*Studies in International Performance*

Published in association with the International Federation of Theatre Research

General Editors: **Janelle Reinelt** and **Brian Singleton**

Culture and performance cross borders constantly, and not just the borders that define nations. In this new series, scholars of performance produce interactions between and among nations and cultures as well as genres, identities and imaginations.

*Inter-national* in the largest sense, the books collected in the *Studies in International Performance* series display a range of historical, theoretical and critical approaches to the panoply of performances that make up the global surround. The series embraces 'Culture' which is institutional as well as improvised, underground or alternate, and treats 'Performance' as either intercultural or transnational as well as intracultural within nations.

*Titles include:*

Patrick Anderson and Jisha Menon (*editors*)
VIOLENCE PERFORMED
Local Roots and Global Routes of Conflict

Elaine Aston and Sue-Ellen Case
STAGING INTERNATIONAL FEMINISMS

Christopher Balme
PACIFIC PERFORMANCES
Theatricality and Cross-Cultural Encounter in the South Seas

Matthew Isaac Cohen
PERFORMING OTHERNESS
Java and Bali on International Stages, 1905–1952

Susan Leigh Foster
WORLDING DANCE

Helen Gilbert and Jacqueline Lo
PERFORMANCE AND COSMOPOLITICS
Cross-Cultural Transactions in Australasia

Helena Grehan
PERFORMANCE, ETHICS AND SPECTATORSHIP IN A GLOBAL AGE

Judith Hamera
DANCING COMMUNITIES
Performance, Difference, and Connection in the Global City

Silvija Jestrovic and Yana Meerzon (*editors*)
PERFORMANCE, EXILE AND 'AMERICA'

Ola Johansson
COMMUNITY THEATRE AND AIDS

Sonja Arsham Kuftinec
THEATRE, FACILITATION, AND NATION FORMATION IN THE
BALKANS AND MIDDLE EAST

Carol Martin (*editor*)
THE DRAMATURGY OF THE REAL ON THE WORLD STAGE

Alan Read
THEATRE, INTIMACY & ENGAGEMENT
The Last Human Venue

Shannon Steen
RACIAL GEOMETRIES OF THE BLACK ATLANTIC, ASIAN PACIFIC AND
AMERICAN THEATRE

Joanne Tompkins
UNSETTLING SPACE
Contestations in Contemporary Australian Theatre

S. E. Wilmer
NATIONAL THEATRES IN A CHANGING EUROPE

Evan Darwin Winet
INDONESIAN POSTCOLONIAL THEATRE
Spectral Genealogies and Absent Faces

*Forthcoming titles:*

Adrian Kear
THEATRE AND EVENT

**Studies in International Performance**
**Series Standing Order ISBN 978–1–4039–4456–6 (hardback)**
**978–1–4039–4457–3 (paperback)**
(*outside North America only*)

You can receive future titles in this series as they are published by placing a standing order. Please contact your bookseller or, in case of difficulty, write to us at the address below with your name and address, the title of the series and the ISBN quoted above.

Customer Services Department, Macmillan Distribution Ltd, Houndmills, Basingstoke, Hampshire RG21 6XS, England

# Community Theatre
and AIDS

Ola Johansson

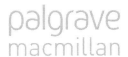

First published 2011 by
PALGRAVE MACMILLAN

Palgrave Macmillan in the UK is an imprint of Macmillan Publishers Limited, registered in England, company number 785998, of Houndmills, Basingstoke, Hampshire RG21 6XS.

Palgrave Macmillan in the US is a division of St Martin's Press LLC, 175 Fifth Avenue, New York, NY 10010.

Palgrave Macmillan is the global academic imprint of the above companies and has companies and representatives throughout the world.

Palgrave® and Macmillan® are registered trademarks in the United States, the United Kingdom, Europe and other countries.

ISBN 978–0–230–20515–4       hardback

This book is printed on paper suitable for recycling and made from fully managed and sustained forest sources. Logging, pulping and manufacturing processes are expected to conform to the environmental regulations of the country of origin.

A catalogue record for this book is available from the British Library.

A catalog record for this book is available from the Library of Congress.

10  9  8  7  6  5  4  3  2  1
20  19  18  17  16  15  14  13  12  11

Printed and bound in the United States of America

*For Amanda, Ezra and Zaza*

# Contents

*List of Illustrations*                                                    ix

*Series Editors' Preface*                                                  xi

*Acknowledgements*                                                         xii

**Introduction**                                                          1
Bringing the messages back to their questions                             7
A festival, travelling troupes, and *ukimwi*                              11
The fieldwork sites                                                       16
Research hypothesis and realization                                       22

**1  HIV Prevention as Community-Based Theatre**                          33
Life as epidemic mimicry                                                  33
The parallel developments of community-based theatre
    and HIV prevention                                                    37
The development of Theatre for Development                                41
The reproductive misfortune of Zakia                                      52

**2  The Performativity of Community-Based Theatre**                      56
Topical uncertainties of traditional practices                           59
The ritual function of speech acts                                        62
The performativity of community-based theatre                            66

**3  The Social Drama of Backstage Discourse and
    Performance**                                                         79
**Part I**                                                                80
    Morbidity and commitment in Ilemera village                          80
    The religious predicament                                            86
    The backstage performance of community-based theatre                 90
**Part II**                                                               92
    The social drama of AIDS statistics                                   92
    The social drama of focus group discussions                          94
    Focus group discussions as action research                           104
**Part III**                                                              105
    A lost performance in Mumbaka village                                 105
    A wider epidemic pattern                                              120

**4   A Deadly Paradox: Assessing the Success/Failure of
     Community-Based Theatre against AIDS**                          **123**
     CBT as epidemiological counteraction                             126
     The multiple lives and deaths of Neema                          130
     Towards a community-based theatre as a relational agency         138
     Recommendations                                                  142

*Appendices*
     Appendix I: Focus Group Discussions: *Modus Operandi*           149
     Appendix II: Questionnaire for HIV Preventive
     Organizations in Tanzania                                        151

*Notes*                                                               156

*Bibliography*                                                        169

*Index*                                                               177

# List of Illustrations

**Pictures**

1   A poster about the increasing burden of funerals in
    Botswana in 2002                                                    2
2   The theatre troupe Red Star rehearsing music before their
    show at the festival in Bagamoyo, September 2001                   12
3   A widow is rescued at the last moment by a neighbour
    as she attempts to commit suicide; performance by Red Star
    theatre troupe in their home town Bukoba, Kagera region,
    in 2004                                                            14
4   The theatre group from the Lumesule youth centre in the
    Mtwara region being transported on the back of a
    pick-up truck                                                      19
5   A ferry on Lake Victoria, close to Bukoba town in the
    Kagera region                                                      34
6   Three female characters perform before an audience in the
    village of Sululu in the Mtwara region                            43
7   A Joker leads a post-performance discussion in the village
    of Sululu, Mtwara region                                          50
8   Audience at a community performance at Bunazi
    market  near the Ugandan border in the Kagera region              69
9   Rehearsal of a scene about circumcision in Mikangaula
    youth centre, Mtwara region                                       77
10  Personnel at the youth centre of Ilemera village,
    Kagera region                                                     80
11  Four women from the village of Gabulanga in an ongoing
    focus group discussion                                            85
12  A young man discusses condom use with counsellors
    in a performance in Birabo, Kagera region                         89
13  A community group performs a dance before the theatre
    performance in the village of Kenyana, Kagera region             129
14  The older brother grabs Neema's hand after demanding
    sex from her                                                      131
15  Audience in the village of Kenyana                                133
16  A woman pushes a man after finding out about his
    second wife; performance in Masasi town, Mtwara region           138

17  A young man presents a plan for a 'youth friendly centre' in
     Muleba town, Kagera region                                              141
18  Mr Andrew Hamisi, a great friend and mentor, was the
     research assistant I worked with most of all during my
     research project in Mtwara region, as well as Dar es Salaam.
     Sadly, Andrew passed away in 2005                                       150
19  Andrew engaged in translation work in Dar es
     Salaam in 2004                                                          150
20  Tanzanian Residence Permit                                              154
21  Tanzanian Research Permit                                               155

## Figures

3.1  Mtwara and Kagera: education (category/topic)                         96
3.2  Kagera: most common topics (per cent)                                97
3.3  Kagera: most common topics among women vs. men                      98
3.4  Mtwara: most common topics                                          99
3.5  Mtwara: most common topics among women vs. men                     100
3.6  General living conditions in Mtwara and Kagera                      101
3.7  General living conditions in Mtwara and Kagera:
      development and recommendations                                    101
3.8  Socio-sexual relations in Mtwara and Kagera                         102
3.9  Gendered proportions of categories in Mtwara and Kagera            103

# Series Editors' Preface

In 2003, the current International Federation for Theatre Research President, Janelle Reinelt, pledged the organization to expand the outlets for scholarly publication available to the membership, and to make scholarly achievement one of the main goals and activities of the Federation under her leadership. In 2004, joined by Vice-President for Research and Publications Brian Singleton, they signed a contract with Palgrave Macmillan for a new book series, 'Studies in International Performance'.

Since the inauguration of the series, it has become increasingly urgent for performance scholars to expand their disciplinary horizons to include the comparative study of performances across national, cultural, social, and political borders. This is necessary not only in order to avoid the homogenizing tendency to limit performance paradigms to those familiar in our home countries, but also in order to be engaged in creating new performance scholarship that takes account of and embraces the complexities of transnational cultural production, the new media, and the economic and social consequences of increasingly international forms of artistic expression. Comparative studies can value both the specifically local and the broadly conceived global forms of performance practices, histories, and social formations. Comparative aesthetics can challenge the limitations of perception and current artistic knowledges. In formalizing the work of the Federation's members through rigorous and innovative scholarship, we hope to contribute to an ever-changing project of knowledge creation.

International Federation for Theatre Research
Fédération Internationale pour la Recherche Théâtrale

# Acknowledgements

In the light of my five-year-long research project there is a range of people and organizations that deserves my sincere gratitude. The Swedish International Development Cooperation Agency (SIDA) was bold enough to give me a research grant that is seldom attainable for scholars in the arts and humanities. Thankfully, SIDA also permitted me to extend the research period of my project as it had to be coped with alongside my new fulltime post at Lancaster University and the birth of a child. Thus Lancaster University also deserves an appreciation. It was, however, the Department of Musicology and Performance Studies at Stockholm University that accommodated my administrative and financial components during the project and therefore I extend a special appreciation to the always supportive Professor Willmar Sauter and the two patient financial secretaries Ingrid Wennberg, and Ann Badlund. I am also grateful for the exciting talks with and Swahili translations by Gachugu Makini at the same department. Furthermore, I extend my gratitude to COSTECH in Dar es Salaam for allowing me to conduct research in five regions in Tanzania.

Palgrave Macmillan editor Paula Kennedy has shown great patience and cooperation with my at times slow production and delivery of results, as have the Studies in International Performance series editors working with the same publishing company, Professors Janelle Reinelt and Brian Singleton. The most patient editorial person was Penny Simmons, however, whose swift work pace I could not keep up with at times but who guided me all the way home through the final proof.

In Dar es Salaam a number of interesting personalities have guided me through various research inquiries. Professor Augustin Hatar, former head of my host Department of Fine and Performing Arts at the University of Dar es Salaam, has been something of a mentor for me as I have studied his profoundly interesting articles, films, theatre performances, and through a number of inspiring talks. Working at the same department is Stephen Ndibalema, a great collaborator and friend whose knowledge and skills in applied theatre has been a continuous source of fascination and motivation. May your wonderful family always be strong!

Furthermore, I am grateful to have met and conversed with Mgunga Mwa Mwenyelwa and Mona Mwakalinga at Parapanda Laboratory Arts.

Three theatre facilitators and researchers at Bagamoyo College of Art were kind enough to share their indisputable experience of Theatre for Development in an interview, namely Professors Juma Bakari, Ghonche Materego, and Herbert Makoye. At UNAIDS/TACAIDS in Dar es Salaam, programme coordinator Henry Meena has been a pivotal catalyst and supporter of the research project. Mr. Meena has a long experience of development work and yet demonstrates a tireless curiosity for innovative and sharp solutions to complex problems in the epidemic. The same can be said about Richard Mabala (previously) at UNICEF, although on as much creative and artistic premises as developmental and strategic grounds.

I am deeply grateful to have worked with a number of research assistants in the Mtwara and Kagera regions in Tanzania. I had the privilege of working with mentioned Stephen Ndibalema during my fieldworks in Kagera 2006. In 2004 I worked with Priscus Kainunula who works for one of the most important civil services for orphans in Kagera, namely Humuuliza. Priscus also offered invaluable help to the CNN team I worked with in the Kagera region in 2004. When I visited Kagera for the first time in 2003, John B. Joseph, programme advisor for Swissaid in Muleba, accompanied me.

In the Mtwara region I am sincerely thankful to have worked with three colleagues, namely Margaret Malenga (2003), Andrew Hamisi (2003 and 2004), and Delphine Njewele (2006). A couple of years ago, I was profoundly saddened by the news that Andrew had passed away. I will always remember his indefatigable thirst for new experiences and willingness to inform me about Mtwara and Tanzania. I will also remember his great parents who invited me into their home and dispensary along the *barabara* nearby Mpindimbi.

Most of all, however, I extend my profound gratitude to the young people in the 20 plus youth/community centres that I visited and revisited in Mtwara and Kagera in 2003–08. I always said it to you and I say it again: you have been directly involved in the most important job in the world and don't let anybody lead you to be believe anything else. Thank you for having accepted my presence before, during, and after performances.

I also feel blessed for having met my greatest critic and love, Amanda.

# Introduction

—What concerns you most about the response to the epidemic today?
—What really concerns me is that while we've made measurable progress on access to treatment, we don't have the same impact when it comes to HIV prevention.

(Peter Piot in his last interview as
Executive Director for UNAIDS, November 2008)

We have all heard the story about AIDS. It has by now become the most devastating pandemic in recorded history. We have also heard about its impact in Africa, a continent that was already encumbered with extreme poverty, undersupplied health services, and slow economic growth prior to the first recorded case of HIV in 1982. And we have all heard about the statistics. More than 40 million people in the world are currently living with the HIV virus – roughly the same amount that has died from the diseases it causes – and of these about 25 million, or almost two-thirds, are living in sub-Saharan Africa.

Tanzania is one of the most AIDS stricken countries in the world, more so than West African countries although less than most countries in Southern Africa.[1] Statistically, Tanzania is an average case in the context of sub-Saharan Africa, which has a median prevalence rate of about 7 per cent. When I initiated my research project in 2003 the commonly referred HIV prevalence rate for the adult population of Tanzania was 8.8 per cent (WHO World Health Statistics 2006: 33). That estimation was recently brought down to a bit over 6 per cent by Tanzania AIDS Commission for AIDS (TACAIDS). The statistical adjustment was due to a different methodological approach to estimated prevalence and

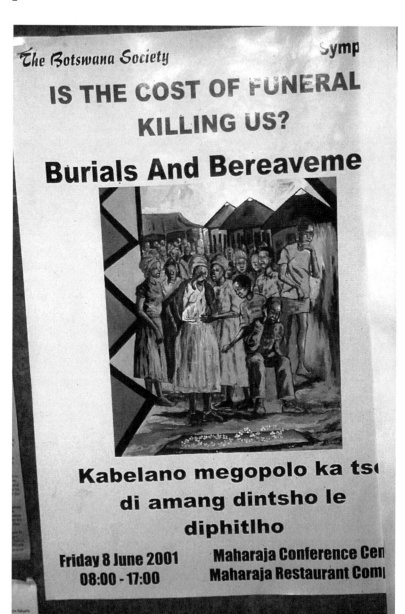

*1* A poster about the increasing burden of funerals in Botswana in 2002 (Photo: Ola Johansson)

incidence rates rather than an epidemiological improvement (NACP report 2008: 5). That is good news for the country, even though any epidemic beyond 5 per cent is considered to be 'generalized' and thus a serious concern to a whole population. Statistics are unreliable, though. The 2005 survey from the Tanzanian National AIDS Control Programme said that 47.4 per cent of all AIDS cases in the country are unknown (NACP report 2006: 2). The same report made clear that about twice as many young women as young men contract the virus in the country. That is probably an overstatement due to a wide margin of error in the estimated data, which to a great extent rely on tests on pregnant women in antenatal clinics. But the overrepresentation of women is, nonetheless, a fact. It is not clear how great the quantitative gender disparity is in Tanzania, but several years' epidemiological surveys have indicated that women in Africa run a greater risk than men of contract-ing the HIV virus (UNAIDS/WHO 2005: 8–9). This epidemic dispropor-tion between the genders was reconfirmed in two recent reports which I discuss further down in this introduction.

Statistics pale in importance compared to direct experiences with individuals. It is enough to see a child such as the young boy I met in a Botswana hospital in Mochudi near Gaborone during a confer-ence on AIDS and literature in 2002.[2] He could not even have his bed sheet rest on his slim body due to the severe state of Karposi's Sarcoma, a skin cancer that makes up a common opportunistic disease of the AIDS syndrome. Around the same time I visited the Grahamstown festival in South Africa and saw the documentary film *Mother to Child* in the series of films called 'Steps for the Future'.[3] The film is about a couple of HIV positive pregnant women in South Africa and their experiences of the existential lottery at a hospital as their newborns will be found to be or not to be infected. The film could not have been more topical as Nelson Mandela, after having failed himself to put AIDS on the agenda dur-ing his presidency in the mid-1990s, started to voice outright criticism against the Mbeki government for its reluctance to roll out programmes with antiretroviral drugs, such as Nevirapine which is the medicine that prevents the transmission of HIV from mothers to children. 'Let the people decide for themselves,' Mandela said and made clear: 'I have expressed that opinion because I believe in it and I am prepared to defend it to the end of my days.'[4] Three years later, the former president would see his oldest son die from AIDS related diseases.

There are more than two million AIDS orphans in Tanzania alone. I remember riding on a motorbike late one night through Bukoba town, the epicentre of the first rampant epidemic on the African continent in the early 1980s, and how overwhelming it was to see the huge numbers of kids roaming the streets around the bus station. They were there in daylight too, of course, but the impression of them in the dark made their vulnerability so distinct.[5] The impression of the orphans in Bukoba engendered a reverse sense about statistics: suddenly the abstract numbers took on a new importance, in virtue of individual cases and social clusters that lead up to the stratosphere of millions. It is not possible to quantify the emotional impact of individuals, that would finish off your sanity pretty quickly, but they yield a concrete need to do something. And so the story that we have all heard of became my own story, prompted by personalized collections of data that indicate a chronic state of living and dying in the parts of Africa I would select as my sites of fieldwork, namely the Tanzanian regions of Kagera and Mtwara.

What, then, can theatre possibly do against the global onslaught of AIDS? The question begs an initial response in terms of perspective. The pandemic is indeed worldwide in reach while theatre can be measured to about an individual's vocal reach. But the global extent of AIDS is merely an accumulation of discrete incidents and therefore a rhetorical construct, which may as well formulate theatre as a global phenomenon if all its varieties and instances are taken together. The epidemiological measurement of AIDS is done through prevalence rates and incidence rates respectively. Prevalence rates indicate, often by highly approximate estimates, the accrued number of cases of HIV-positive people in a certain area. Incidence rates indicate the frequency of infectious transmissions over time in certain areas. It is thus the prevalence rates which make up the masses of cases behind the statistics, while the frequency of incidences pertain to series of individual cases. In order to understand the qualitative matters behind the quantities of cases it is inevitable to attempt to appreciate the rationale behind individual incidents in the pandemic. There cannot be an incident that occurs in a larger situation than the reach of, say, a voice. In most cases the infection is transmitted through human contact. That is as theatrical as anything can be.

'Awi!' a leader of a theatre group shouts within that vocal scope, and an audience responds with a collective 'Awa!'. It is then reversed: 'Awa!' – 'Awi!'. It is like testing a communal microphone on a traditional meeting ground to see if it still works. All public events in rural Tanzania oscillate in the diachronic continuum of traditional practices and contemporaneous modes of performance and there is no given agreement between the poles. Urbanized young spectators may openly mock shows that appear obsolete, while people from rural elder communities can do the same at progressive performances. That is the first auspicious premise of community-based theatre: it is a highly mobile and challenging phenomenon which cuts through cultural layers of time and space as well as demographic and generational differences. Far from theatre institutions or educations, most forms of local perform-ance can be said to be maximalist in their mixed means of oration, drumming, dancing, singing, storytelling, poetic recitations, dramatic dialogue, and post-performance discussions in the interactive sphere of performers and spectators. And when the groups start up an event with *ngoma* (Kiswahili for drum-based dance), many people still come gather-ing and often respond spontaneously by joining the performers.

Theatre of this kind readily alters between registers of style, aesthetics, and vernacular. If there is a way to bind the presence of a space with the memory or genealogy of an audience, initiatives will be taken to perform such visions, as, for instance, through the ritual dance *Omutoro* in the Kagera region. The latter ritual dance-theatre stems from a past royal tradition of reporting back to the king about battles in the field, by way of a confrontational choreographic style accompanied by stan-zas that sound like contemporary rap music. In the age of AIDS, the depicted battles are transposed to narrative attacks on wholly different scenarios about plebeian rather than royal affairs. A similar diachronic performative statement can be found in the other region of my project, the Mtwara region, where a mime enacts a tacit protest against the mul-tiple use of one and the same knife in boys' circumcision ritual (*jando*), whose secrecy is breached in favour of the need to break through a cul-ture of silence. In these and many other cases discussed in the book, the alteration between traditional practices, long-established aesthetics, and local languages meet the need of a present-day crisis which cuts across taboos, secrecies, and tacit cultures in Tanzania. Without the backing of applied community-based theatre from the African continent, however, it would probably not be nearly as efficacious.

Community-based theatre is indeed the most site-specific cultural practice used against AIDS in Tanzania today, but if its local adaptability has to do with malleable and exchangeable elements, its overall eclectic concept is international and even intercontinental. It started out in the mid-1970s as Theatre for Development (henceforth abbreviated TFD), a label I will avoid in the book due to its monetary overtones and its typical one-time task-based project format. Apropos definitions, Cohen-Cruz writes:

> Thinking of theatre and development so broadly evokes various modes of 'applied theatre' that have circulated since the late 1960s. Applied

theatre is the array of practices that assay to ameliorate situations through such means as building positive identity and community cohesion through the arts. Take, for example, community-based theatre, a popular mode allied with identity politics and targeting under-represented groups in quest of collective expression. While related to TFD, there are important differences. Community-based theatre is partisan, dealing with a particular group: TFD is bi-partisan, dealing with a particular population AND a 'civil society' institution.[6]

However, in my opinion TFD is almost always engaged in a specific developmental task, while CBT is about addressing an entire society's way of life. In appearance and planning CBT has a lot in common with TFD, but its undertaking is always about overall lifestyles and longitudinal social patterns, often without a clear and discrete objective in sight. This kind of project and performance practice has also been called Theatre for Social Change, but, as will be clarified in the first chapter, the objective of CBT need not only or primarily be about education, development, or change but may be about a scrutiny of or attention toward concealed and tacit living conditions. TFD, a culture-historical extension of instructive dialogues by colonial representatives and, after the independence of several African nations in the 1960s, pedagogical dramas by post-colonial playwrights and facilitators (Kerr 1995), was elaborated as an experimental form of adult education in the 1970s (Kidd 1973). Under the influence of Paolo Freire and Augusto Boal, theatre workers in countries like Botswana and Nigeria started to blend the traditional arts and meeting forms with contemporary techniques of participatory pedagogy and dramatic performance. In Chapter 1, three phases of applied theatre are outlined along with a cognate development of HIV prevention forms. Pre-written touring theatre shows distinguish the first phase; the agenda-driven and task-based TFD typifies the second phase, while CBT exemplifies the third phase. It is in particular the third phase of applied African theatre that comes to the fore in this book. A number of intracontinental meetings and workshops during the 1970s led to an application of theatre through which mobilized social groups themselves took on the planning, organization, analysis, script-writing, rehearsals, performances, evaluations, and follow-up projects. CBT is a serious attempt in favour of people's ownership over their traditional practices, intellectual properties, aesthetic styles, and, *in extenso*, current private and social affairs.

Even if CBT entails the label 'efficacious theatre', its functional features do not ensure a successful outcome of, say, an increased awareness of AIDS if, to be efficacious, a successful outcome requires a translation of awareness into practice. (I remember thinking about this every time the bus passed by a biblical quote on a building in Mwenge en route to the University of Dar es Salaam: 'Every promise needs performance.') One of the findings of the study will divulge that CBT as a form of HIV prevention lies so close to the epidemic determinants of AIDS that it is reasonable to assume that if a well-conducted CBT project fails, for example, through a communicative breakdown between performers and spectators after performances, lack of political follow-up initiatives after the revelations of a performance, and so on, it is probably not only a problem of the theatre or the project format but also the epidemic determinants of AIDS. CBT is performed by the very same cohorts that are most susceptible to HIV: young people without wealth who are often required to meet other people's demands in order to make their own ends meet. A failure among these young people can very well be indicative of precisely why HIV spreads in a culture of silence or corruption or power imbalances in a certain area. It may also be the case, *mutatis mutandi*, that a project which turns out to be seemingly efficacious may be quite useless after its completion. Countless pilot projects in Tanzania and other African countries affected by AIDS intervene in schools or other controlled settings, bringing with them packages of information about AIDS as a social and medical syndrome, holding a meeting with teachers and pupils, testing the information material on pupils by way of a questionnaire or something similar which the young ones respond to accurately, and then reports are sent to the overseas home office about the success of the project along with an additional note about the need for further funding. It needs to be said that such projects can be useless and without any effect whatsoever. The reason for this is, again, that the failure and success of HIV/AIDS prevention in most places in Africa is not about lack of information, education, or medication, but about the possibility to renegotiate historically regulated lifestyles.

## Bringing the messages back to their questions

My first thoughts of a research project on African theatre against AIDS came into view at a theatre festival in Bagamoyo, Tanzania in the fall of 2001. At the time I had just started a post-doctoral position at Stockholm University, besides holding a freelance contract as a theatre critic with the daily paper *Svenska Dagbladet*. When I suggested writing an article about the festival in Bagamoyo for the paper, the editor of the culture section said it was a great idea so long as I did not expect any compensation on top of the ordinary pay for the text and pictures. Swedish papers do not send out critics or correspondents to cover theatre festivals unless they take place in Avignon, Edinburgh, or Berlin. But I already had the journey funded by the prize money that I had been lucky to win the previous year for my doctoral dissertation at Stockholm University.

By coincidence I had a couple of interesting shows to review the week before I took off. One was Bernard Koltes's *Back to the Desert* at the Royal Dramatic Theatre and the other was Jean Genet's *The Blacks* at Stockholm City Theatre. Both plays had built-in thematic connections to Africa, but I was particularly excited about the latter with its visiting performance by South African Market Theatre since I was familiar with the reputation of the legendary Johannesburg company. The experience did not turn out as I expected though – in fact, I barely remember seeing the show at all. The date was the 11 September 2001 and when the lights went up on stage all I could think about was the jet liners that flew into New York's Twin Towers killing thousands of people. When I arrived in Dar es Salaam four days later, I found an edgy political climate with street demonstrations in anticipation of the upcoming election that year. I also became aware of a public opinion, at least among young adults on the buses to and from the university, which spoke of an America that had brought 9/11 upon itself. At this point, just a few days after the events in New York and Washington, everybody was talking about Osama bin Laden and al Qaida. It may seem odd that people in Dar es Salaam of all places would even come close to tolerating bin Laden's actions; his first major terror plot was after all executed in Nairobi and Dar es Salaam only three years earlier. The bombs were directed at American embassies and many more people had died in Kenya than in Tanzania, but the casualties were almost exclusively Africans and the rationale and methods of the deeds could hardly be justified by anyone. But the reaction in Tanzania, like many other places outside the Northern hemisphere, has to do with other things than specific facts in contemporary plots. A major blow to the core of a superpower by a fringe rebel movement is perceived as a quite sensational and heroic act in a country that has been subjugated for centuries by foreign slave traders, colonial imperialists, Cold War superpowers, and global agencies and corporations.

Later on in September 2001, I became engaged in readings and discussions about another catastrophe: AIDS in Africa. This was a much slower tragedy and one whose sensationalism took much longer to put into perspective. Like everyone else I had once associated 'African AIDS' with truck stops along murky roads where crowds of prostitutes established shantytowns with names but with no location on maps. In an article published in 2001 called 'Killer on the Road', Kevin Toolis writes about one such place on the highway between Kenya and Uganda called Salgaa where 300 prostitutes invite truck drivers to stop for sex:

> Inevitably, Salgaa and the other truck stops like it are an engine of an epidemic; an amplifier of the Aids holocaust that has infected an estimated 14 per cent of Kenya's population. The trucks barrel down the highway carrying tea to Mombasa, machinery to Uganda, exotic flowers and vegetables to Nairobi for overnight airfreight to Europe. They also carry the Aids virus circulating in the bodies of the drivers and their assistants. But blaming the men for buying sex is naive and simplistic. Many Kenyan drivers spend two weeks on the road driving in harsh conditions and sleeping in squalid hotels. Inevitably, some men will, through drink, loneliness or lust, buy themselves sex – and some comfort – on their endless journeys across the African savannah. It's not sex, commercial or otherwise, that is killing Kenyans, but a tiny piece of genetic material, the HIV virus. Trying to change private sexual behaviour is almost impossible.[7]

I remember reading articles like these and sensing a resemblance with adventure stories from wild and exotic places outside the law. Toolis uses the word holocaust, while many other journalists and commentators make comparisons between AIDS and the plague ('black death' is, of course, a favourite simile), warfare, and other spectacular analogies. This is not surprising in the light of the enormous death toll associated with AIDS; in sub-Saharan Africa alone the syndrome kills twice as many people as the 9/11 tragedy every day. It is just that the apocalyptic analogies risk standing in the way of an understanding of the actual causes and effects of the epidemic if their rhetorical impact takes over the motifs of reports or, indeed, political speeches. In his article, Toolis goes on to say that it is understandable to buy sex when you are spending weeks on end on the road as a truck driver and that it is not, after all, sex or the prostitutes that kills them but the virus. Toolis also points out that changing behaviour, despite the fact that 'everyone in Kenya knows about Aids', is 'almost impossible'. This is where the article needs to be called into question. It is hard to fathom a holocaust attributable to a virus without holding fully aware carriers of the virus responsible. It is understandable to have sex on the road under alienating working conditions, but it is not reasonable to have sex without responsibility (i.e., protection) given an understanding of the risks involved. This 'private sexual behaviour' is an act with life-threatening consequences not only for the truck drivers and prostitutes but also other sex partners as well as the spouses and children of the drivers and sex workers. Hence, under the given circumstances, sex can hardly be perceived as a private act, if it ever could.

Only later did I realize that it is scenarios in a much more mundane reality that actually drive the epidemic. I got a strong suspicion of such a scenario when I read a different kind of article, namely in the Dar es Salaam based newspaper *The Guardian* (and its weekend edition *Sunday Observer*) right before the festival in Bagamoyo:

> A total of 93 teachers in Dodoma Urban, Kondoa and Mpwapwa districts in Dodoma Region have died of AIDS since September last year. The Dodoma Regional Chairman of Tanzania Teachers Union (TTU), Abel Maluma, said deaths caused by AIDS related diseases had been on the increase in the region, affecting academic performance in the area. According to statistics, out of the 93 teachers who have died, 52 came from Kondoa District and six from Mpwapwa. Maluma said that Dodoma Rural District, whose statistics were not immediately available, had lost the largest number of teachers to AIDS. He said most of the victims were female teachers who he said were being used as sexual machines to entertain public officials who visit their areas. Maluma said one of the reasons why the disease was spreading among the teachers was due to the fact that most of them do not practise safe sex. He said TTU in the region had started a campaign to educate the teachers on how to avoid the disease, lest they all perish.[8]

The Tanzanian *Sunday Observer* is not a sensationalist tabloid, nor an anti-governmental newspaper, it simply reported this story as a simple *fait accompli* in a rural district of the country. I remember being shocked over the tiny cameo strip in the margin of the paper's inner section. Ninety-three teachers in one region in one year? Had it been sex workers along a murky route in East Africa it would have been comprehensible, but teachers used as concubines for public officials in the same district as the country's capital?[9] I wonder if it was possible at all for these teachers to raise the awareness of their pupils about sexually transmitted infections while being used as call girls for politicians and other very important people. And how can politicians expect teachers to be role models if they are not even allowed to play the role of themselves? The predicament in the Dodoma region exemplified a moral double bind since it appeared to be at once both an official affair and confidential routine. Many people, from the grassroots all the way up to governmental headquarters, are outspoken in private and quiet in public about these kinds of affairs. Exactly that crossing point between public and private issues is a site to explore for applied community theatre. So how can the theatre negotiate the double bind in its capacity as cultural event? Perhaps the Bagamoyo festival could offer a clue?

## A festival, travelling troupes, and *ukimwi*

The five-day festival at the Bagamoyo College of Art offered a range of interesting types of performing arts from most Tanzanian regions as well as some international places. Students from the college presented a mixed bag of stylistic abilities in a performance that depicted AIDS from downright hilarious to doomed scenarios. Some dance performances were hypnotizing; gigantic drums carried on the heads by performers from Burundi were beaten so hard that the whole town's soundscape trembled; there were acrobats that made me seriously worried about the health and safety of the performers; and there was choir music that pitched inspirational passions alongside profound dirges about the epidemic, the *zeitgeist* of the country, and the future of its children.

The host troupe, Bagamoyo Players, put on a strong performance called *Wewe na Mimi* ('You and I'). It was about a woman called Mofa, who becomes stigmatized by her employer, her boyfriend, and her family respectively when it is established that she suffers from AIDS related diseases. It proved to be the first of many performances with similar themes on stigmatization. A wide variety of additional themes were also spotlighted at the festival, such as the use of condoms, promiscuity, polygamy, circumcision, widow inheritance, orphanhood, money, witchcraft, ignorance, and nonchalance. Just to organize a several day long festival on AIDS is, of course, an important statement in itself. At a closer look, however, it was really more than a statement in the literal sense of the word, for most performances went beyond their enunciated objectives by saying that speech is not enough and that action must follow upon every word. In an extended sense, then, the act of looking at the shows involved a tacit pledge that implied doing what one can to prevent further harm and loss.

As soon as I thought of commencing a research project on theatre against AIDS I decided to direct my attention to its preventive capacity,

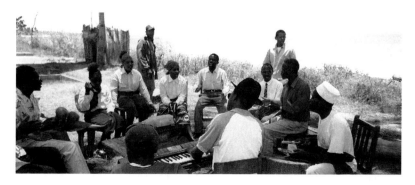

2   The theatre troupe Red Star rehearsing music before their show at the festival in Bagamoyo, September 2001
(Photo: Ola Johansson)

as opposed to its informative, explanatory, illustrative, or invocatory depictions. Many people and texts repeated the same thing over and over: as yet there is no model or practice of HIV prevention that has proven efficacious. Just as many people and texts, however, spoke of theatre as a great mobilizer and catalyst for preventive actions for young people, who make up the most vulnerable cohorts of the epidemic. It seemed clear that cases worthy of note would be such where the theatre goes up against genuine challenges of AIDS control, to the point where it proves to be either efficacious or ineffective. Only one full-length book had been written on the subject at that point, namely Marion Frank's doctoral dissertation *AIDS Education through Theatre: Case Studies from Uganda* (Bayreuth: Bayreuth African Studies, 1995). The book explored early types of campaign and festival theatre in the 1980s, very much in line with what I saw at the Bagamoyo festival and which will be described in Chapter 1 as the second phase of theatre for development.

Most of the performances at the Bagamoyo festival exhibited scenarios which one could either sympathize or disagree with. One show divulged a peculiar conflict beyond its scripted dramaturgy though. It was not necessarily the best piece of the festival, but what made me curious about the show by the company called Red Star from Bukoba was an unexpected occurrence towards the end of their performance. It occurred at a high-pitched intrigue in which a brilliant comedy actor portrayed an elderly man who ran into a series of misunderstandings in company with younger women. Since my Kiswahili was nonexistent at the time and since I could not always hear what my fellow interpreter was saying, I could not quite grasp what happened on stage, let alone what transpired between the performers and the spectators. A whole section of the audience suddenly became noisy, some left the arena, while numerous remaining spectators continued to throw comments at the stage throughout the show. Verbal remarks from the audience are very common in African theatre and a vital and dynamic quality of live performances, but in this case I sensed an almost hostile atmosphere in the audience. The day after, I found the leader of the group, Michael Kifungo, and asked him what had happened the night before. With an embarrassed smile he explained that the Bagamoyo audience, which is more urbanized than their own audiences in Bukoba in the north-western corner of Tanzania, did not approve of the way the group depicted crude misunderstandings about things like condom use.

It is of course an advantage as well as a limitation of festivals to accommodate visiting performances that pertain to spectatorial views elsewhere. I took an interest in the Bagamoyo festival not as a self-contained event, but as an entry point to a theatre whose place and function I had to follow back to from where it came. Many groups at the festival were travelling troupes with ambitions to become professional or semi-professional companies. I certainly enjoy watching the repertoire of travelling theatres and have nothing against their commercial aspirations, but they do not meet the optimal interest of the research in this book, which has to do with the function of community-based theatre (CBT). Before I go into detail about the latter form of theatre and my fieldwork, I will describe my acquaintance with some travelling companies that helped me to define the research project.

In Bagamoyo I promised Kifungo that I would travel to Bukoba and see his company perform theatre on its home turf sooner rather than later. Since then we have in fact met several times and become close friends. Kifungo's group operates in an area whose modern history has been drastically shaped by the AIDS epidemic. With great flexibility, they can travel from fishing communities on Lake Victoria to interior agricultural villages to provisional market places with one and the same play, adapting the plot to the respective target audience and their local context. Sometimes during such journeys, I imagined that this must have been what the post-Independence travelling theatre of the 1960s felt like, both playing and seeing.

The strongest piece I witnessed by Kifungo's company was a play about a woman who loses her husband to AIDS and thus all her belongings in the 'property grabbing' that ensues after his death. This form of cultural and personal misfortune is quite common for widows in

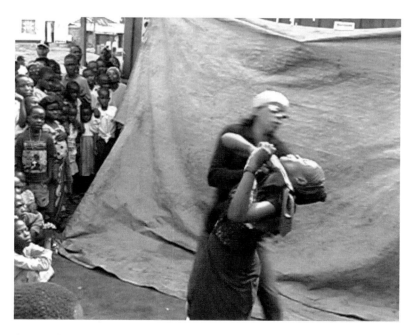

*3*   A widow is rescued at the last moment by a neighbour as she attempts to commit suicide; performance by Red Star theatre troupe in their home town Bukoba, Kagera region, in 2004
(Photo: Ola Johansson)

the Kagera region and a frequent theme in performances on AIDS, as will become clear below. Kifungo himself, arguably one of the greatest comedy actors in Tanzania, again enacted an old man who personifies promiscuous lifestyles of old, preferably with younger women. He even hits on a nurse in a hospital scene who works for a doctor who has just informed him and his family about the risks of HIV. The performance I captured on video, and have subsequently used in several lectures and seminars, took place near a major intersection on the outskirts of Bukoba town. If the group took on a challenge with the urban audience in Bagamoyo, this was no less daring. The loud cacophony of the nearby traffic culminated in a collision between two lorries, which stole the attention of the audience for a moment, but the company managed to draw them back into the drama. Audiences in market places and other public spots are restless and on the move, but in this case Kifungo and his company made at least a hundred people stand still for almost an hour thanks to a performative register of intensity suggestive of comme-dia dell'arte. The remarkable turn of the performance, however, came towards the end of the show when it all turns to something as uncommon as a tragedy.

The husband is dead and buried, the widow is emotionally heartbroken, materially ruined, and probably also infected by the virus that will bring her to a slow and painful death. So she attempts to do something that is frequently spoken of behind the scenes of the epidemic reality, but almost never performed in scenes of African theatre: suicide. With a scarf as prop the woman puts the rope around her neck and is about to fall to her death when a neighbour runs into her house and saves her. A doctor is called in to support the miserable woman and he arrives at the same time as the same extended family that deprived the bereaved woman of all her belongings. The doctor says that there is hope for AIDS widows (even though this was before the distribution of anti-retroviral medicines in Bukoba and Tanzania), that she should go to the Kagera regional hospital down the road, get a test done, and that there is a free counselling service. The doctor then turns 90 degrees on his heel, while delivering his informative lines, away from the woman to face the audience. He asks if they recognize what they have just seen and if they have gone for a test. 'What about you?', someone responds from the audience. The challenge takes the actor by surprise and all he can do is to return the question: 'Na wewe ye?' In the next moment Kifungo re-enters, now in ordinary clothes, and takes up a well-known song about the perils of AIDS to which the rest of the group responds in the mode of a gospel choir. After the song Kifungo takes over the role as Joker by recapturing the key themes of the performance and then turn them into a participatory audience discussion.[10] He invites people to comment on specific characters for the purpose of making the comments and questions direct and concrete. The post-performance discussion turns out well and gives several spectators a chance to speak out. Everybody gets reminded about something that must never be forgotten and that must turn from discourse to practice, or, put differently, from rehearsal to performance at the end of the day.[11] The difference in atmosphere and response could not be greater from that which the group experienced in the amphitheatre of Bagamoyo the year before.

Well-performed travelling shows can be very imposing and entertaining and lend themselves perfectly to the camera lens. That is partly why I instantly suggested revisiting Kifungo's troupe in Bukoba when the television network CNN offered me the chance to produce a short documentary film about theatre against AIDS in Africa.[12] However, I wanted to do more than just make a stunning display of the opportunity. First of all, I decided to have no voiceover, but let Kifungo and a female co-performer do the talking. Second, I wanted to include scenes of condom use from performances since Kifungo's group was brave enough to promote contraceptives against the official agenda of his group's patrons, namely the Evangelical Lutheran Church (ELCT) of Tanzania.[13] Third, I realized that the CNN piece would not make a difference on the ground in Africa unless I actively brought the production down to an interpersonal and communal level. Therefore I introduced the coming broadcast by email to development organizations and aid agencies that I knew held a vested interest in Tanzanian HIV prevention. Some of them reacted positively to our film and maybe, just maybe, the television feature made it a little easier for Kifungo's group to land a long-term contract with a major international donor organization the following year. In the film, we also showed the previously mentioned warrior dance called *Omutoro* performed by an orphan group who substituted the old belligerent lyrics with stanzas about the contemporary enemy called AIDS.[14] Moreover, we interviewed regional AIDS coordinator Dr Mussa at Kagera Hospital. He described the frustration as a doctor of seeing people die (i.e., in the fall of 2004 about a year before the first antiretroviral medicines were allocated to the region), but he also expressed his conviction that applied theatre can be an effective means against AIDS. Regrettably, the latter comment never made it through the final cut of the documentary.

It is clear that many people invest heavily in modern media rather than traditional modes of communication such as live community performances. For the present research context it needs to be said that to employ television, video, newspapers, the internet, and other new media for HIV preventive purposes is out of touch with the experience of most rural people in Tanzania where most HIV positive people (in absolute numbers) reside. Very few people among the most susceptible strata have access to modern media. While radio is completely dominant when it comes to electronic mass media, the best chance of communal intervention is still through interactive performance. No participant among the theatre groups I have studied in the Kagera region saw the CNN piece, except those who I notified and who went to public places such as bars to see the broadcast. Hence the TV production functioned more or less like a communal performance for those who got invited by the producer of the show.

## The fieldwork sites

In 2002, I revisited Tanzania to look into the possibilities of conducting a meaningful research project down there. At that point I relied on advice from two individuals in Dar es Salaam. One was Agustin Hatar, at the time head of the Department of Fine and Performing Arts at the University of Dar es Salaam, who had written a series of highly sig-nificant field reports and essays from applied projects that he had led. Hatar suggested that I visit a paralegal group that he had trained in the region of Morogoro. It turned out to be a very rewarding first visit to a group who put their own living conditions and its connections to AIDS in play. I visited a rehearsal of a new play outside the group's counsel-ling office in Morogoro town. It started with a choir for the purpose of giving the occasion an inviting atmosphere and mobilizing people to the performance site. A group member told me that she wished they could summons people by drum-based dances, like people do in places like Mtwara region in southern Tanzania, but Morogoro does not have such a repertoire of drum-based dances.[15]

In the performance a schoolgirl becomes pregnant by a fellow stu-dent, but she does not know which one until she takes a test which indicates a boy who also happens to be an intravenous drug addict. The girl also shows signs of illness. The girl's parents become devastated when notified about the pregnancy and ill health, to the point where the father threatens to beat the mother for her leniency toward their daughter. After some convincing the father agrees to join the mother and daughter for a counselling session. On recommendation by a female friend, the mother decides to consult the locally based Faraja Trust Fund since they combine diagnosis and counselling. The latter organization is an actual partner of the theatre group in Morogoro. At once I noticed the difference of 'being there', within the field of refer-ences in the presence of a theatre whose messages are intended to be acted upon, as opposed to the remoteness of the appeals at the festival in Bagamoyo the previous year. Just like Kifungo's group in Bukoba, the paralegal group in Morogoro oscillated between naturalism and comedy with a good amount of improvisation to boost both styles. The father refuses to even get close to the daughter in a way that brings out laugh-ter, despite the harshness of the paternal attitude. His hostile stance is about to spill over into ferocity as he gets the message that his daughter has contracted HIV. Again, he threatens his wife physically. The father had thought that it was a matter of tuberculosis (TB) when it actually turned out to be AIDS. (TB is the most common cause of death for AIDS patients in Tanzania, so the girl *could very well be* suffering from the disease, which is part of the range of opportunistic diseases of the syndrome called AIDS.)[16] The counsellor manages to calm him down and he eventually accepts the situation. What remains after this intense intermezzo is a brief epilogue by the counsellor, who emphasizes the importance of caring for HIV positive people in a loving manner. She then leaves the subject open for audience discussion.

The other person who advised me on an entry point to an eventual research project was Henry Meena, programme associate at UNAIDS, who suggested that I look into the conditions of community theatre and HIV prevention in Mtwara region as a comparative geographical example to more established activities in the Kagera region. Both sites turned out to be decisive for my project. It was only natural to make the Kagera region one of the comparative sites of fieldwork. This is the region where the country recorded its first AIDS case, namely in Ndolage hospital on the hilly slopes of Muleba district in early 1983, just a few months after the continent's first case had been recorded across the border in the Ugandan Rakai district. Kagera is a coffee and banana producing region with a fishing industry as it is situated on Lake Victoria. The region does not have critical food shortages but this well-being is eclipsed by the fact that it also has the lowest GDP per capita in Tanzania. Kagera borders Rwanda and in connection to the genocide in 1994, along with the continuing warfare in Burundi, the Kagera region has received almost one million refugees. The ensuing social instability and personal insecurity makes parts of the region unsafe to travel through and I have personally been on some stretches where a police escort has been necessary. Kagera also has a long history of sexually transmitted infections (STIs) and high infertility rates after serious syphilis epidemics in the 1930s and 1950s (Killewo 1994). The determinants behind the historic epidemics as well as the contemporary AIDS epidemic make up a combination of cultural and biological rationales. The region, especially with its largest ethnic group called Haya, is a patrilineal area where the economy has been controlled almost entirely by men and where women have long had a national reputation of prostitution, most likely due to a heavily unbalanced gender division of labour (I account for this in greater detail in Chapter 1). Another contributing risk factor in the AIDS epidemic is that the region exemplifies a very low rate of male circumcision (Hanson 2007: 6). Kagera is, moreover, a region with lots of functioning theatre groups under the aegis of various non-governmental organizations (NGOs) and governmental AIDS coordination, which makes it an interesting comparative case to the less prolific theatre region of Mtwara. In Kagera I have conducted research in two districts, namely Muleba and Bukoba rural.

In Mtwara region, in southeastern Tanzania with borders to the Indian Ocean and Mozambique, I have also carried out fieldwork in two

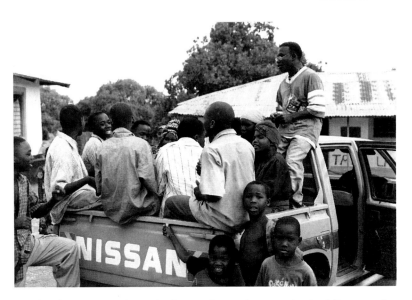

*4* The theatre group from the Lumesule youth centre in the Mtwara region being transported on the back of a pick-up truck
(Photo: Ola Johansson)

districts, Masasi and Mangaka. Small-scale farming dominates the districts, with cashew nuts and simsim as major cash crops. It is considered to be utterly poor and inaccessible even by Tanzanian standards. A book presents the geographical area as follows: 'This corner of the country is officially one of the poorest corners of the world and is always presented as a peripheral area' (Seppälä and Koda 1998). A socio-economic report puts it even more bluntly: 'The southern zone as a whole and Mtwara in particular is unattractive to the new generation who move out in search of greener pastures elsewhere in Tanzania. They are economic "refugees". To stem this outflow means a lot of work in making the region and the zone economically attractive to young people' (*Mtwara: Socio-Economic Profile 1997*: 29). Seppälä describes the geographical remoteness of the region well:

> The relative isolation of the southern regions needs to be placed under closer scrutiny. First [...] the sense of isolation is increased by the fact that on all sides the immediate neighbouring areas are equally poor and marginalized. Thus short-range trade and interaction does not function as a substitute for poor communication with

Dar es Salaam. Second, the physical characteristics of the surrounding areas make the area more isolated. The area is bordered by uninhabited forests in the north and the Indian Ocean in the east. The barrier of forests in the north functions as a frontier not just in real terms but also in the formation of perceptions. When one enters the area from the north by car, one travels for several hours through the wilderness, interrupted by a few small settlements. The dominance of nature over human construction is striking. Thus the existential experience of a traveller is like a rite of passage: first you leave one situation, then you are thrown into a frightening transitional phase and only when you have passed through it are you initiated into a new situation.

(Seppälä and Koda 1998: 12)

Even though the region has a fairly dense population, its population growth rate is the lowest in the country (ibid.: 10–11). Even colonial personnel tried to steer clear of the area and it is said that the unpopular ones down the ranks got stationed in Mtwara. There are researchers who believe, on good grounds, that the population growth will stay low,[17] but the trend may in fact turn upwards in the near future due to a major infrastructural reform programme in the so-called Mtwara corridor, linking the interior parts of East Africa from Zambia and Malawi to the harbour in Mtwara town, and, not least, linking the region with neighbouring Mozambique by means of a proper bridge. Up until now, one has had to enter the bordering country by small boats, or even by wading in the dry season, across the Ruvuma river.

The marginality of Mtwara may appear to be quite obvious today, but the region has been subject to pivotal events in the history of Tanganyika (former mainland Tanzania). Masasi district is located along the Arabian slave route that reached from the ancient harbour of Kilwa to the area of Malawi. The Maji Maji uprising against the German colonizers took place here in 1905, which has its most renowned depiction in Ibrahim Hussein's drama *Kinjekitile* (1974). One ethnic group from the Malawi area who allegedly were on their way back home after escaping the slave traders in Kilwa remains in Masasi, namely the Yao (or Wayao in Kiswahili plural). Other ethnic migrations have brought the Makua and, to a lesser extent, the Makonde, with their widely celebrated wood carvings, from Mozambique to Masasi. As usual when it comes to the division of tribes, it is important to remember that such an 'invention of Africa' (Mudimbe 1988) with reference to the ethnic labels 'have been given as a by-product of the colonial administration and research' (Seppälä and Koda 1998: 28).

The mentioned ethnic groups, along with a smaller number of the Mwera, were traditionally organized in matrilineal societies, meaning that, for instance, marriages entail:

> the husband's moving to the wife's premises, and the children are named after the woman's brother, the maternal uncle who is responsible for important rituals and ceremonies and has to be informed of them before they can be arranged. The bride wealth is handed to him when the sister's daughter gets married and he is responsible for bringing up the sister's children.
>
> (Shuma 1994: 174)

These are observations of matrilineality among Mwera by Shuma (1994), but they may as well be ascribed the other mentioned groups – or, at least they probably could in the past. Today the kinship systems are far from intact and may be characterized as a demographic-historical bilineal hodge-podge after ethnic displacements, interethnic marriages, colonial interventions, superimposed national laws and regulations, and current lifestyle changes. The gradual disintegration of social organization has had a very detrimental impact on women and youth, who 'fall in between the systems in many different ways' (Swantz in Seppälä and Koda 1998: 175; Shuma 1994). The collapse of defined social roles has had an even more damaging effect on vulnerable groups since AIDS entered the geopolitical scenario of the Mtwara region in 1986. Concrete cases of this will be described and analysed below, not least in connection to a performance from Likokona village. While a positive aspect of the interrelated ethnicity is its relatively peaceful coexistence; there are religious tensions, especially between some Christian and Muslim factions. As always in Tanzania, however, there is a tacit agreement hindering tribalistic or ideological interests from developing into violent conflicts. Land conflicts are more serious than clashes over politics or religion (Seppälä and Koda 1998: 195–221). It is perhaps pertinent to describe the interethnic relations in Masasi in terms of Mbembe's post-colonial discourse, which supplements the dichotomy of resistance and collaboration by what is called 'illicit cohabitation' (Mbembe 1992: 4).

The traditional societies have been radically remodelled by intervention of world religions like Islam and Anglican and Roman-Catholic branches of Christianity, as well as superimposed socialist programmes such as the so-called *ujamaa* ('villagization' in translation) scheme whereby villages were uprooted and forcibly moved into greater farming

communes in locations that were meant to, but seldom did, offer sufficient means for a sustainable livelihood. This political leap combined
with periods of drought has created regular bouts of food shortage and
famine in Masasi.[18] These aspects and many more will become important parts of the subsequent discussions of theatre and its deployment
against HIV/AIDS.

### Research hypothesis and realization

My research project was motivated by an initial hypothesis which
had the following convoluted phrasing: Given that the most critical
problems with AIDS have to do with communicative taboos, social
predicaments, and gender troubles for young, poor, rural people that
existed before the biomedical syndrome of HIV/AIDS, it ought to be fair
to assume that CBT is an auspicious, and thus potentially efficacious,
mode of HIV prevention since it is primarily organized and performed
by young, poor, rural people, and that it is very popular, and that it has
built-in problem-solving techniques, and that it uses traditional as well
as contemporary means of social mobilization, interactive practices,
and follow-up programmes. The hypothesis pointed to correspondences
such as the following:

- Young women and men are the prime risk groups in the AIDS epidem-
  ics of Tanzania as well as many other parts of sub-Saharan Africa.
- More than 50 per cent of the sub-Saharan population is under 20.[19]
- In many rural places, CBT offers the only means of critical discourse
  on AIDS and public opinion for young people.
- It is extremely popular in Tanzania (as well as many other sub-
  Saharan countries).
- It is in line with state-of-the-art HIV prevention philosophies.

The question is not, however, what theatre can do to counteract AIDS
so much as how realistic it is to assume that something communicative,
social, and gender oriented can be fulfilled in the politicized, religious,
and conservative conditions of Tanzania. CBT is about much more than
a breakthrough in a culture of silence. CBT is about the preparation,
organization, and performance of HIV/AIDS scenarios that are seldom
or never spoken of, let alone acted upon in order to be thrashed out in
communal post-performance meetings. I would go as far as to assume
that CBT is about exemplifying the very conditions of local AIDS epidemics insofar as it coincides with its social and performative *modus*

*operandi*, through the ones who are at greatest risk.[20] The book explores the potential efficacy of CBT as an eclectic form of HIV prevention in Tanzania, with a few additional references to comparable sites and activities in Africa. The exploration entails research into assessments of community-based theatre (performance analyses), epidemiology (area studies and interviews), ethnography (culture-historical accounts of the areas in question), and young people's shared and private experiences (focus group discussions and interviews). Examinations and correlations of both official top-down and communal bottom-up approaches lead to decisive interpretations of culture-specific epidemics, HIV prevention schemes, and the relational functions of theatre within such frameworks. The diachronic links between contemporary CBT, traditional practices and communal meetings, as well as the hybrid associations of theatre, popular culture and art, everyday discourse, and internationally developed methods of participatory performance make it possible to compare CBT with performative functions in political speech, formal ritual, and informal communication, as well as various forms of HIV prevention.

The book is written in three successive chapters which lead up to a fourth chapter where the limits and prospects of CBT against AIDS are evaluated. Each of the three 'explorative' chapters assumes a special angle of approach towards the hypothesis that was mentioned above. Moreover, all chapters exemplify case studies which epitomize their thematic orientations respectively. The first chapter is about the corresponding developments of community-based theatre and HIV prevention. The second chapter compares the eclectic qualities and functions of CBT with the invariable forms and authoritative mandate of ritual by comparing their potential efficaciousness through the concept of performativity. As it turns out, the HIV prevention schemes of the first chapter and the ritual regimens of the second chapter have trouble reaching and bringing out the 'backstage reality' of the epidemic. The third chapter takes into consideration such backstage factors by weighing the official accounts of HIV prevention and the ritual legacy against focus group discussions and interviews with the 20 theatre groups and village dwellers residing close to the groups. The research hypothesis, based on the modal assumption of CBT's qualities as potentially efficacious means of HIV prevention, is thus driven into three blind alleys that all end with a variation of the following paradox: despite the fact that CBT arguably meets more 'best practice' criteria than any other form of HIV prevention;[21] and despite that it can be perceived as more ritual than initiation rites and rites of affliction under contemporary living conditions; and despite that it actually brings out the backstage discourses and practices in critical and participatory ways, it may not be possible to assess, let alone ascertain, its efficacious facility as HIV prevention. There are a couple of rationales behind this paradox. First of all it is, and will always be, impossible to ascribe or estimate a specific measure of success to a discrete practice in a complex situation (like an epidemic) in which efficacious actions require several concurrent and coordinated schemes. Second, it is my conviction that CBT can only attain its optimal cogency or influence if it is openly and legitimately backed by political and other authoritative advocates.

Chapter 1 introduces the performative and epidemic scenarios in the Kagera region. The chapter describes retrospective developments where increased epidemiological pertinence and democratic representation in HIV prevention as well as community theatre eventually brought the two forms of actions together in the 1990s.[22] HIV prevention programmes and applied theatre started out as expert driven activities in Africa, but gradually had to adhere to local knowledges and lifestyles. Three successive phases of African community theatre are outlined: (1) the travelling theatre of the 1960s; (2) the theatre for development movement of the 1970s; and (3) contemporary modes of community-based theatre which were established during the 1980s and that have been enhanced since then. The parallel trajectory in HIV prevention is more recent but similar in its successive phases and kinds as it went from: (1) white-collar KAP (Knowledge Attitude Practice) studies in the 1980s; (2) NGO sponsored IEC (Information, Education, Communication) campaigns in the 1990s; and, finally, (3) community-based programmes, often in the name of BCC (Behaviour Change Communication) and sometimes aligned with inclusive multi-sectoral and 'mainstreamed' schemes, in recent years.

In Tanzania, Penina Mlama, Amandina Lihamba, and Eberhard Chambulikazi from The University of Dar es Salaam lead the way to topical community-based theatre projects around 1980, which meant that the planning, performance practices, and follow-up components of projects were gradually handed over to local residents, even if the latter were initially facilitated by artistic outreach workers and supported by external donors. A case study signals a warning, however, already in the first chapter of the book. A seminal theatre project facilitated by Mlama in 1982 is analysed in detail, with the result that a state-of-the-art community project on the reproductive health conditions for young women right around the epidemic outbreak of AIDS in the neighbouring region of Kagera did not differ essentially in either themes or outcome from most of the present-day theatre projects against AIDS. One explanation of this matter is coincidental; many of the risk factors behind AIDS are generic insofar as the determinants of the syndrome share various characteristics with cognate sexually transmitted infections as well as related social problems in terms of, for example, gender inequities. However, the fact that a theatre project on the sexual conditions for young women almost three decades ago functioned and ended in the same manner as contemporaneous theatre projects against AIDS also indicates a problem with the use of theatre.

In response to the predicament of generalized use of community-based theatre, I argue that projects do not always adapt enough site-specific features in current and epidemic conditions, which has to do with, first, obsolete notions about the function of community theatre stemming from the days of agenda-driven and task-based TFD projects predicated on, and aiming for, rapid change and/or a self-reliant group interest as a means in itself, and, second, with Western cognitive notions of individual behaviour change by the organizations that deploy and fund outreach theatre. The combined fallacy has left many theatre groups physically isolated and psychologically defeatist. There are, of course, exceptions and I will devote as much interest to auspicious initiatives as critique against flawed ones.

The predicament is analysed further in the second chapter.[23] The new complex challenge of AIDS necessitates a fresh view and deployment of community-based theatre. The reconsideration is motivated by specific comparisons with traditional practices, such as initiation rites and traditional health practices, but also contemporary outlets, like alternative prevention practices and public political discourse. In this chapter a variety of performance practices that underpin community-based theatre are considered. In Tanzania, like many other sub-Saharan countries, rural people still gather when they hear the cue for meetings in the form of drumbeats and local dances (*ngoma*) in public hubs. Audiences enjoy choral songs (*nyimbo*), poems (*mashairi*), and acrobatics (*sarakasi*) as well as theatre (*michezo ya kuigiza*) in numerous stylistic and aesthetic registers.

In Mtwara region the initiation rites for male (*jando*) and female (*unyago*) youth are still defining gender roles to the detriment of domesticized women. These rites are compared with the initiation rites called *Nkang'a* (female) and *Mukanda* (male) of the Ndembu that Victor Turner analysed, again with less attention to the relatively submissive formation of social female identities. In Mtwara, the average age for initiates has gone down from 13 to below ten years, which is indeed detrimental for the health of children and youth. The theatre, controversially, reveals secrets from initiation rites when necessary, for example, when young people's lives are at stake due to the multiple use of blood-stained knives in male circumcisions, or when old fashioned educations on sexuality and marital conduct carry on anachronistically for young women. In both regions of the study, far more people go to traditional doctors than modern health facilities for treatment, also with AIDS related opportunistic infections and diseases.

When it comes to comparisons with alternative prevention schemes, it is by now clear, as mentioned earlier, that one-way communicative modes of information such as TV and other audiovisual media has a limited influence on young people in both regions since so few have access to such outlets. Some youth centres that I have visited have been given video players and information tapes from donor agencies, but in Tanzania almost all people are by now aware of the essential information about HIV/AIDS as a health risk. An exception as regards modern media is the wide ranging and much less expensive radio, through which, for instance, hip-hop artists (playing so-called *bongo flava*) in Tanzania have proven to take great responsibility as role models in terms of depictions of AIDS. Radio can also be used as an interactive component if people gather round broadcasts and then discuss and even act upon or re-enact shows, which was what the organization CARE did in Ethiopia when I was there in 2003. Such community initiatives, as well as the CNN feature I took part in, are covered under my definition of community-based theatre. However, what is needed today, rather than media campaigns, is inclusive projects involving interpersonal life skills in sexual negotiation backed by income-generating activities, gender-balanced household economies, and a political support that becomes known in whole districts and regions. This is where the social mobilization, transethnic familiarization, participatory methods, and public interactivity of community theatre come in.

Political speeches have proven to be deficient if enunciations remain isolated from pragmatic efforts on the ground. Many leaders have talked about the 'war on AIDS', but never identified who the enemy is. A more serious aspect of political speech is when it implicates a hidden religious agenda, despite the fact that religious dogmas consistently contradict the National Policy on AIDS (2001) in Tanzania. The gap between rhetoric and deed lends itself to a discussion geared by the concept of performativity. The comparison concentrates on the mode of influencing interpersonal or societal changes through speech and other modes of action (rather than simply knowledge, information, education, or communication). Traditionally social scientific dichotomies have ascribed performative functions of social change to ritual, while theatre has been degraded to serve as entertainment, reflection, and statement. However, apart from the fact that the latter dichotomy is categorically flawed, culture-historical changes, partially due to AIDS as such, have altered the functions of cultural practices. Community-based theatre is a more interactive, variable, adaptable, and democratic forum than traditional rites and can be said to hold possibilities of contemporary 'ritual changes' for HIV preventive purposes. I show this by site-specific examples of community theatre as an eclectic type of performance with diachronic and syncretistic qualities from the continuum of formal ritual (initiations, circumcisions, dances, etc.), semi-formal communal meetings (political speech, church choir songs), and informal everyday life (scenes of domestic life, risk behaviours in public spheres). Hence the predicament identified is not a necessary flaw of community-based theatre as HIV prevention *per se*, but has rather to do with a narrow understanding of AIDS as a modern societal syndrome and, moreover, of a questionable attitude to theatre as a democratic mode of public opinion and life skills.

Methodologically, it should be clear that I have no direct part in the theatre activities I am studying, but in fact try to minimize the reactive effects of my presence among the informants. This matter is, of course, worthy of a study in its own right and cannot be exhausted here. I have worked as a teacher in community, political, and educational theatre at Lancaster University (2005–09) and performed in a few productions, although not in Africa. A recurrent mode of study is performance analysis with the cultural and interdisciplinary scope pertaining to performance studies and epidemiology. Hence the analyses of performance may be described as studies in an extended field of methods and references. The examples are mainly taken from my fieldwork sites in Tanzania, but also from a few other African countries.[24] I start with quite common examples of community theatre, where it breaks the silence on the epidemic, depicts taboo-laden situations in public, and involves audiences in post-performance discussions. In particular, more contentious performances that challenge the communicative and political limits of public events are examined. A few case studies from both corners of the country lead the way. One is taken from Likokona, where a woman gets disinherited by her own brother, despite living in the matrilineal belt of southern Tanzania. She takes the case to court but is framed by inconsiderate politicians, a corrupt judge, and defeatist community members. The Likokona performance is highly controversial, which may turn out to be counterproductive in its conservative context and thus indicative of the limits of CBT as public opinion and political instrument.

The book investigates a field of extended performative practices where three scopes of epidemiological studies are correlated, namely (1) official versions of the epidemic; (2) the theatre group members' version of the epidemic; and (3) the site-specific depictions of the epidemic in theatrical performances. The first aspect is by now thoroughly researched by epidemiological studies of the countries in Africa and the districts in Tanzania, even if the Kagera region is much more mapped out than the Mtwara region. The second aspect has been dealt with by means of focus group discussions (FGDs) and interviews with 20 theatre groups in Tanzania, which are modes of activities that are treated as performances in their own right in Chapter 3. The third aspect has already been mentioned in terms of an extended discourse of performance analysis.

My contribution to a more generalized study of official attitudes and opinions on AIDS is to keep track of the relations of themes among the groups I am analysing in performance but also by conducting semi-structured talks. The distribution of topics that group members themselves propose for focus group discussions reveal culture-specific inclinations and, not least, gender-specific preferences that make me look upon statistics as an interpretive material. I devote the first part of Chapter 3 to the explication of statistical relations, which in turn is a pre-stage to the performance of focus group discussions. A decisive step towards a fuller assessment of the efficacy of theatre against AIDS is to interpret so-called backstage situations and their relations to front-stage versions of the epidemic, that is, what is enunciated and enacted behind closed doors and in public respectively. As discussed in the second chapter's comparative typology of performance variants, CBT does the opposite of initiation rites, namely it turns social order inside out by familiarizing taboos that are being defamiliarized in public. Focus group discussions and interviews behind the scenes, as presented and evaluated in Chapter 3, divulge sensitive revelations about religious, ritual, political censorship, and a defeatist attitude towards the gender tragedy of having many more young women exposed to HIV than men through transactional sex.[25]

The taboo-laden backstage performances often relate indirectly to CBT. What is said in private is not always enacted communally but underlies metonymic scenarios that audiences are let in on surreptitiously or through other forms of dramatic allusion, or just by appealing to conscious local residents. Focus group discussions (FGDs) and interviews with theatre groups and spectators/villagers offer exclusive insights to various risk situations. After a performance about the communal stigmatization of an HIV positive man, a focus group discussion with young women in Mumbaka stagnates from the start as they giggle in embarrassment over the silence. But my FGDs are based on topics suggested by the interlocutors themselves. I ask them to mention the three most precarious risk factors when it comes to HIV in their community. My tactic is to await responses to the proposed topics, even when silence reigns for a minute. In the presence of a shy group, I either start with an easy topic (usually related to the epidemic implications of poverty), or else take a chance and start with a peculiar topic. In Mumbaka I asked about a topic that was suggested by one person only, namely rape. Eventually a young woman crossed the narrative threshold and cautiously told a story about how men regularly come up to unfamiliar women along the road and demand sex, with little or no possibility for women to say no. Eventually all women join in the discussion and revealed a range of critical risk factors caused by gender inequity that may lead to violent incidents.

In most cases FGDs and interviews confirm that community performances actually dramatize the most sensitive issues in the epidemic. Every so often, however, I have discovered discrepancies in the relation between, for example, epidemiological surveillance reports in a certain area and the discursive representations of AIDS among people, or between performances and backstage talks. No quantifiable, discursive or performative mode of communication is privileged in my study, but they are rather compared with one another in order to consolidate a shared epidemic reality against which to work out interpretations and recommend follow-up actions. Some stories are incredible in their own right as individual statements. Most stories support the notion of gender problems as the root cause behind the cross-cultural epidemic determinants.

After seeing African CBT for six years and formalizing fieldworks for four years I can say with confidence that my project gravitated towards the conclusion that gender predicaments are generating the most prevalent epidemic determinants, even behind such disparate cultural regimes as the clan systems of the Kagera region, the matrilineal kinship systems of the Mtwara region, the fishing industry demographics around and in Lake Victoria on the border to Uganda, and in rites of passage in societies along the Ruvuma river on the Mozambique border. Everywhere I go, see, listen, and analyse public as well as backstage performances there are striking gender inequalities in play. This was recently reconfirmed in a report from the World Health Organization (WHO 2009) and the statement after the fifty-fourth session of the Commission on the Status of Women by the Joint United Nations Programme on HIV/AIDS and the United Nations Development Fund for Women (UNAIDS/UNIFEM 2010). The WHO report established that AIDS is now globally, 'the leading cause of death and disease in women of reproductive age' (WHO 2010: 43).

> Globally, women represent about 50 per cent of all people living with HIV, and over 60 per cent of HIV infections in Africa. In Southern Africa, prevalence among women aged 15–24 years is on average about three times higher than among men the same age. [...] Gender inequality and discrimination, including violence against women and girls, are a key driver of women's and girls' increased vulnerability to HIV infection and to the disproportionate impact of the epidemic. This is further exacerbated in situations of humanitarian crisis. Mobile populations also often become vulnerable to HIV. We know that lack of economic, social and legal autonomy of women and girls limits their capacity to refuse sex or to negotiate safer sex and to resist sexual violence and coercion, including transactional sex and early forced marriage.
>
> (UNAIDS/UNIFEM 2010: 2)

Most of these risk factors will be exemplified and analysed in the chapters ahead. Rather than merely stating 'what we know', however, CBT and its backstage social dramas also offer viable ways of counteracting risk factors. That is the difference between the social science of epidemiology and the practice-based research of performance: the first observes, calculates, and makes analytical inferences while the latter observes, analyses, and acts out interpretable key incidences. This book is an attempt to combine the merit of both the social scientific and the performative approach to HIV prevention.

The most widely stated risk factor in performances I have seen, among people I have talked with, as well as in official reports, is undoubtedly poverty and its links to sexual lifestyles. This generic rationale carries comparative possibilities to past epidemics of sexually transmitted infections in a global perspective, which in turn prompts an important disclaimer. There is no reason to believe that AIDS is a primarily *African* predicament, just as there is nothing particularly African about the sexual habits that spread the virus. One good way of testing the validity of myths is to turn one's attention to one's own circumstances. In the latter part of the nineteenth century, Sweden had a comparable economic standard as Tanzania has today and similar patterns of syphilis epidemics as Tanzania has with AIDS epidemics today. Stockholm had the highest rates of sexually transmitted infections (SDIs) among

European cities and just as with serious levels of AIDS, outbreaks of syphilis indicate a social condition in which more men than women had casual and transactional sex, while the ensuing SDIs, and especially the then deadly syphilis were embedded in a taboo-laden culture of silence (cf. Holmdahl 1988). The myth about an 'African sexuality' (Arnfred 2004) as a cause of AIDS has been disproven, for example, in terms of a so-called coital frequency in epidemiological studies, which show a similar regularity of sexual intercourses pretty much all over the world (Caldwell and Caldwell 1996; Pickering et al. 1996), Tanzania included (Konings et al. 1994).

Politicians, academics, NGO workers, urban feminists, teachers, religious leaders, and community people know that AIDS is driven by gender imbalances, but they are also aware of the fact that women have gone through a series of revolutions in social and political status in various parts of the world. With an apparent risk of victimizing Tanzanian women, which can only be mitigated by referring directly to African women's own discourse and actions, besides justifying it through feminist and postcolonial discourses, an inevitable outcome of my studies is to report the fact that being a housewife is the most hazardous position to occupy in contemporary sub-Saharan Africa (excepting that of being under five years old with the risk of contracting malaria). The most common type of HIV incidence is quite undramatic, namely marital sex in family households. Two general, and often overlapping, scenarios dominate the epidemics: either mobile men bring home the virus via more or less established extra-marital affairs (associated with epidemic patterns in southern Africa), or women engage in transactional sex, not seldom to support their children (associated with certain epidemic factors in eastern Africa). Within one and the same household moderate and extreme poverty may coexist, again in favour of men. Poverty is not only too generalized a concept to translate and apply in prevention programmes, but also as an ethnographic premise for interpretation. Hence gender, not poverty, is the lowest common denominator in my understanding of AIDS in the areas of study, or, put differently, the interpretive plot closest to the ground which most pertinently captures various local facts and values in a way that makes it possible to do something about.

In the forth and final chapter, an accumulation of arguments based on case studies in previous chapters sustains my decisive interpretation of gender predicaments with special attention to post-performance commitments and (a lack of) follow-up programmes.[26] If applied theatre is assessed as a relational means of action research within the framework of aligned prevention schemes rather than, quite naively, as a means in itself or a means for rapid social change, or as a means to simply deliver messages for health promotion, there are viable grounds for a theatre with real impact and sustainability. In the light of the tripartite correlation of official, communal, and private perspectives toward the epidemic through the combined methodology of epidemiological studies, performance analyses, focus group discussions, and interviews, the attempt of the study is to evaluate the efficacy of HIV prevention through theatre. In virtue of my findings, I put forth a few best-practice cases and attempt to vindicate their worth by demonstrating a culture-specific relevance, an ethical soundness through gender-balanced organization, a cost-effective feasibility by means of their voluntary basis and social mobility, and a commitment by young people to organize epidemiologically relevant counteractions. It is thus my goal to go beyond, on the one hand, anecdotal evidence and, on the other, far-fetched cultural interpretations and instead combine macro- and micro-perspectives in order to substantiate a realistic and applicable concept of efficacy when it comes to CBT as HIV prevention.

# 1
# HIV Prevention as Community-Based Theatre

AIDS became known in the Kagera region in 1983 and in this geographical location it is fair to assume, in virtue of correlations between outreach projects and statistical data, that travelling theatre troupes in conjunction with community-based theatre groups have had a certain impact on declining mortality rates, from a devastating quarter of the population in parts of the region some twenty years ago to a few odd per cent of the general population today.[1] In this chapter, I will discuss the capacity of theatre to counter the epidemic challenges by offering a culture-historical retrospective of the epidemic as perceived in performances, and later by approaching contemporary quests for HIV prevention through a discussion of efficacious CBT. In order to show what HIV prevention and community-based theatre are up against, it is important to avoid a simple narrative about 'AIDS in Africa' and instead identify by way of concrete examples the many AIDS epidemics in the region and indeed in Tanzania as well as other parts of the world.

## Life as epidemic mimicry

AIDS epidemics disseminate like global economies across cultural boundaries and national borders, incognito and yet intimately incorporated in peoples' metamorphoses from local to global ways of living. The syndrome took on epidemic proportions in central Africa and in the urban centres of the North American coasts about the same time. Before that it is reasonable to suppose that it had meandered up the Congo basin to the highlands of Rwanda before reaching Lake Victoria on the border of Uganda and Tanzania where large numbers of people fell ill in the early 1980s. There are good reasons to assume that the source of the epidemic is to be found in western equatorial Africa, due to the vast range of viral subtypes detected in that area (Iliffe 2006: ch. 1). It is assumed by many experts today that the human immuno-deficiency virus (HIV) originally 'jumped' from simian species (carrying SIV, simian immunodeficiency virus) to humans in Cameroon, where it is not uncommon to hunt and eat chimpanzees.[2] However, since the virus is constantly changing, the challenge to understand how and where it spreads and to prevent that incidence rate is of much greater importance than to know where it came from.

When HIV became an epidemic in the Kagera region it was alien to everyone. A macabre spirit sneaked into people's lives like a myth from nowhere and haunted them seemingly by quirks of fate, took possession of their bodies, one by one, invisibly, hollowly, silently, until wearing them down in a slow, unbearable loss of life. Despite complex epidemio-logical surveys, it is still hard to know where AIDS came from, where it is going, and how to prevent it from getting there. The syndrome is generally acquired in sexual relations and causes a set of symptoms to transpire through quite familiar ways of living and dying.

The distinctive features of HIV as a virus were that it was relatively difficult to transmit, it killed almost all those it infected (unless

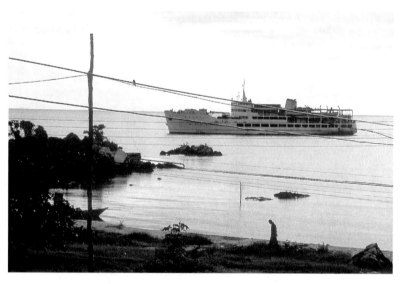

5   A ferry on Lake Victoria, close to Bukoba town in the Kagera region (Photo: Ola Johansson)

kept alive by antiretroviral drugs), it killed them slowly after a long incubation period, it remained infectious throughout its course, it showed few symptoms until its later stages, and when symptoms appeared they were often those common to the local disease environment. This unique combination of features gave a unique character to the epidemic, 'a catastrophe in slow motion' spreading silently for many years before anyone recognized its existence.

(Iliffe 2006: 58)

AIDS was and still is a 'ghost disease' (Hanson 2007a: 28), which has gradually come to be recognized via corporeal signs that bear various taboo and stigma laden code names, sometimes with sexual overtones (Mutembei 2001: ch. 4). An informant in southern Tanzania portrayed an inconvenient truth about the ominous ghost with a Kiswahili aphorism: 'umekaa pakunoga', roughly meaning that it is 'situated in a delicious place'. AIDS is a performative double that imitates people's lifestyles – it does what people do. It travels with people, stays in their houses, goes to rendezvous with them, has sex with them, has kids with them, becomes sick with them, and dies with them. Apparently, AIDS has no traceable origin or fixed identity, it shadows people and mocks scientists in an epidemic mimicry – just like syphilis, the 'great imitator' of old – whose transmutations can only be pursued and interpreted in the nomadic choreography of changing locations, identities, and lifestyles.[3]

In Africa, cultural changes have been historically induced by geographical and violent political circumstances. The continent is in many areas sparsely inhabited, which means that people have always had to travel long distances for various purposes. Low population density makes services arduous and costly, curbing an effective health care system.[4] The geographical predicament was intensified during the long history of the slave trade which displaced ethnic and demographic groups, and through the colonial division of labour as male workforces were allocated to distant production sites while women were left behind in village households (Barnett and Whiteside 2002: ch. 5; see also Iliffe 1995: 269–70). The gender disruptive colonial order, with spouses absent from each other over long periods of time, caused a number of epidemics of sexually transmitted infections (STIs) and has been one of the crucial causes behind the rapid spread of AIDS in sub-Saharan Africa. In more recent times, women are carrying out considerably more work than men in

Tanzania and other parts of Eastern Africa, while men still control the household economy and hold the outreach function of selling and buying merchandise.

On and around Lake Victoria in the beginning of the 1980s the historical traces of AIDS were among fishermen, lorry drivers, and blackmarket racketeers involved in the so-called *magendo* economy (Barnett and Blaikie 1992: ch. 5), who unknowingly carried the looming epidemic further into Africa via truck stops, bars, and marketplaces populated by penniless local women offering transactional sex. A few years later, a similar transnational epidemic emerged in southern Africa, where contact between prostitutes and migrant workers such as miners would threaten about a third of the adult populations in countries like Botswana, Zimbabwe, Swaziland, and South Africa.

Early in the epidemic, people in Kagera region suspected witchcraft and incriminated the Ugandans (and vice versa). They refused to believe that they got fatally ill from having had sex a decade ago, shunned the sick like the plague (which it was), and were wary of conspiracies among modern doctors with their useless 'international' medicines. Political leaders declared war on AIDS, but never identified the enemy.[5] Religious leaders blamed people for amoral promiscuity, but could not avoid contracting the virus themselves. Health researchers eventually held a retrovirus responsible, but offered no hope for a cure. At the end of the day the authoritarian speculations, advice, and judgments meant little, and so people on the ground had to look for more precise and pragmatic questions and solutions amongst themselves. Within a few years in the 1980s, the epidemic became generalized in many parts of Tanzania and East Africa, that is, with prevalence rates exceeding 5 per cent in adult populations. The syndrome cut through the social fabric of ethnicities, interests, sectors, and social strata; the major risk groups were no longer sex workers and truck drivers, but traders, farmers, teachers, students, politicians, clerics, housewives – in short, each and everyone. By 1990 it was obvious that AIDS was much more than a health issue. Yet most governments, including the Tanzanian, delegated the lion's share of their preventive resources to the health sector. This deferred an adequate response by about ten years. Not until New Year's Eve in 1999, when about one in ten Tanzanians were infected, did president Benjamin William Mkapa declare AIDS a national disaster in a speech (TACAIDS 2003: 10). Since then there have been genuine attempts to address the immediate epidemic concerns, even if the discursive openness and political willingness has mostly been manifested on a national rhetorical level, while the coordinated responses by governmental agencies at district and village levels have been much less open and efficient.[6]

## The parallel developments of community-based theatre and HIV prevention

By delineating the parallel developments of community theatre and HIV prevention, the reciprocal needs of the practices will become quite evident and be assessed in the light of certain case studies. Tanzania has taken a leading position in the implementation of sustainable and locally owned theatre projects, but the challenges of AIDS have proven so vast that previously supposed purposes of community theatre must be called into question. Rather than being viewed as a means in itself, or a means for rapid change, CBT will be considered as a relational means in coordinated programmes against AIDS. However, in spite of functioning as an exceptional relational agency for the most exposed cohorts in the epidemic, the social, gender, and epidemic predicaments will persist as long as policy-makers do not fully recognize the status of young people and the capacity of community theatre.

Some phenomena are so big that they need to be made smaller to be fully comprehended. The global implications of AIDS rupture any conceptual definition and cultured imagination. It is now clear that it is the most devastating epidemic in recorded history and that it continues to plague populations in sub-Saharan Africa who struggle with extreme poverty, societal discontinuity, and scanty health services.[7] Yet the substance of the epidemic is found in a drop of blood, semen, or even a tear.[8] Reducing the epidemic to microscopic sizes, however, brings discourses into a *mise-en-abyme* of medical taxonomy. To grasp the practical issues of AIDS, a halfway point of view needs to be established, from which the macro-statistics and micro-samples coalesce in life-size interactions. Coincidentally, that perspective involves scenarios about as big as a theatrical production from a performance researcher's point of view.

In the light of the complex pathological make-up, social secrecy and sexual taboos, I have found CBT to be more expressive than clear-cut medical information on HIV and AIDS, more accurate than epidemiological statistics, and more relevant than scientific analyses of its causes and effects. The syndrome, which few talk about but most people cannot help but watch when acted out, is a communicable disease primarily in the social sense of the word. Its routes of transmission are statistically estimated in vast incidence rates, but theatre shows just how complicated one such incidence is for affected people.

Medical prevention research approaches the syndrome objectively, but the lack of a cure 25 years into the epidemic performances show how biased the impact of AIDS is, especially for young women and widows. It is more dangerous to be a housewife than a soldier in Africa. In some parts of southern Africa, young women are up to five times more likely to contract HIV than men. In Tanzania, the gender inequity is slightly less striking in statistical terms but still highly significant in real-life situations. These are statistical facts that have been verified consistently over the past five to ten years (cf. UNAIDS/WHO 2004; WHO 2010; UNAIDS/UNIFEM 2010). Theatre is the mode of testimony and dissent that reveals such complex, biased and inequitable conditions on a community level and, as long as it is not fully recognized by policy-makers, community theatre will continue to fail as no other HIV prevention dare fail.

In what follows I will provide a brief historical background by showing how HIV prevention schemes and CBT projects have been developed in parallel and gradually converging trajectories, from top-heavy, expert-driven campaigns to bottom-up approaches increasingly owned and run by community residents. After that it will become clear what a pivotal role theatre can actually play in HIV prevention. But just as the virus has an eerie ability to evade a medical solution by mutating, neither discrete nor generic preventive practices are sufficient in the complex and heterogeneous epidemic. In the light of past and current cases in Tanzania, I will suggest that CBT can make a difference in an advancing epidemic only if its own *modus operandi* is open to culture-specific variations of the epidemic. Seen as a relational means of change rather than a means in itself, or a means for rapid imposed change, theatre against AIDS can be fully appreciated and applied as a participatory prevention practice in an epidemic that ultimately hinges on social interactions rather than pills or money.[9]

Catherine Campbell poses fundamentally complex and difficult questions about the social impetus of the epidemic in her acclaimed book *'Letting Them Die': How HIV/AIDS Prevention Programmes often Fail* (2003): 'Why is it that people knowingly engage in sexual behaviour that could lead to a slow and painful premature death? Why do the best-intentioned attempts to stem the tide of the HIV epidemic often have so little impact? To what extent can local community mobilization contribute to a reduction in HIV transmission?' (ibid.: 183) Quite naturally, Campbell does not have ready answers for her radical questions. The reason for this is simply that there are still more questions to test than answers to apply on the syndrome. The major challenges concern the gap between knowledge and practice among general populations. How is it possible to prevent life-threatening behaviours among people who are aware of the risks (how HIV is transmitted), situations (where and when it happens), means (how to protect oneself), and consequences (the slow and painful death) of AIDS? The most troubling thing about this question is perhaps not that it is still unanswered, but that it took such a long time to pose to people who may hold answers. Instead of asking questions, so-called experts and aid workers for a long time brought what they thought were answers to affected people, while it should have been the other way round.

HIV prevention campaigns in sub-Saharan Africa were for a long time predicated on biomedical information and rational-choice theories pertinent to Northern societies (Freudenthal 2002). Models such as the theory of reasoned action (Ajzen 1980), the health belief model (Conner and Norman 1996), and social learning theory (Ormrod 1999) are all based on generalized ideas on how individuals attain preventive conduct through cognitive, observational, or behavioural skills, intended to predict positive outcomes of future decisions. The favourite methodology for the models comprises surveys conducted after certain doses of information, sometimes mixed with heuristic exercises to inculcate the achieved knowledge. In the 1980s particular risk groups' knowledge, attitude, and practice (KAP studies) were mapped out, followed by a distribution of pamphlets and other mainly written material in information, education, communication (IEC) campaigns. The most renowned example in the 'invasion of acronyms' (Nugent 2004: ch. 8) is the World Health Organization's ABC model, spelled out as abstain, be faithful, use condom.

The problem with the generic prevention models is that HIV transmissions can seldom be avoided by virtue of individual decisions or discrete behaviour. It does not really matter what you know or opt for if you do not know who your partner last had sex with and if it is considered unsuitable or even unsafe to ask about it, even if he suffers from a noticeable sexually transmitted infection and you are not in a position to say no to sex, or propose to use a contraceptive, since that would make him suspicious of whom you last had sex with, which may well be a legitimate concern as that affair may be your only chance to put food on the table for yourself and your children while your husband is away working, or looking for a job, or spending time in his *nyumba ndogo* ('little house', a metonym for mistress in Swahili).[10] Even if this scenario – pointing to some of the most common routes of HIV transmission in sub-Saharan Africa today – involves stock characterization in a seemingly foreseeable plot, its preventive *raison dêtre* cannot be boiled down to a level of individual decision making in a controllable setting. Geopolitical, cultural and ethnic variations must always be taken into account as they involve gender roles in social systems that have likely developed in other places, times, and circumstances than the present. This is one of the crucial challenges in HIV prevention schemes, namely the double-edged understanding of the culture-historical backgrounds of various ethnic groups and, correspondingly, the way their cultures have been geographically displaced and structurally disintegrated over time (Barnett and Whiteside 2002: ch. 5). Some of the driving forces behind gender imbalances and generational clashes lie embedded in the historical and political discrepancies of pre-colonial, colonial, and post-colonial times. The question is how to cope with them in a viable way today. This is, as will be clear below, where the diachronic and eclectic praxis of community theatre enters the epidemic scenario.

In the 1990s prevention workers gradually realized that HIV and AIDS are not merely a medical, moral, or behavioural challenge, but a syndrome which cuts through the cultural fabric of whole societies. Prevention programmes were thus designed to incorporate cultural underpinnings and local participation in behaviour, culture, communication (BCC) campaigns based on interactive processes and tailored messages through a variety of communication channels to effect individual as well as communal behaviour changes. In recent years community programmes have turned former objects, or 'target audiences', of projects into collaborating and ultimately self-reliant subjects, a 'paradigm drift', as it were, from expert information to grassroots participation (Campbell 2003: 9).

Hence the answer to the question of why people knowingly engage in life-threatening sexual behaviour has little to do with risk factors as such. Solutions must be pursued beyond abstract categories like 'knowledge', 'attitudes', and 'behaviour', which are only effects of underlying causes. The degree of risk-taking implicated in the spread of HIV relates to social groups lacking a livelihood which would allow them to make safe choices in life. The most vulnerable group, women aged between 15 and 24, is trapped in a vicious circle where the lack of resources often leads to interrupted schooling, early marriages, and pregnancies, and ensuing transactional sex. According to the most recent statistics in Tanzania, 47.4 per cent of all AIDS cases are unknown (NACP Surveillance Report 2005: 2) and many more women than men are tested (primarily in antenatal clinics), but the existing data, nonetheless, speak volumes about gender-specific susceptibilities.

Among the cumulative AIDS cases in the country between 1987 and 2004, 1.6 per cent of males aged between 15 and 19 were found to be infected, while the same age cohort for females reached 4.5 per cent. Among males aged between 20 and 24, 7.4 per cent are estimated to be HIV-positive, while the rate for women is 16.5 per cent (NACP Surveillance Report 2005: 3). When it comes to absolute numbers of people living with HIV or AIDS in the period from 2000 to 2006, the estimated number is 40,000 for males aged between 15 and 24 and 100,000 for females of the same age. The same statistics for persons aged between 20 and 24 indicate that 80,000 men versus 220,000 women are infected (ibid.: 45). A similar gender deviation is found in surveys of infections transmitted sexually, the main physical cause of HIV transmission. About twice as many AIDS cases come from married couples than single people (ibid: 6). These statistics disprove previous notions about AIDS as a medical problem among certain risk groups engaged in certain risk behaviours; rather, the data says that AIDS is a generalized syndrome that reveals social issues, in particular for female strata, that have been around for much longer than the epidemic itself and have to be coped with by means of culturally inclusive and integrated prevention schemes. Community theatre takes on a crucial place in HIV prevention with regard to the mobilization of young people, gender-balanced programmes, and a communal examination of traditions through past and present cultural practices.

## The development of Theatre for Development

With the acknowledgement of local knowledge as an untapped resource for HIV prevention programmes, a mixed practice of culture-specific conflict- and problem-solving leads into the AIDS scenario: CBT. African applied theatre, signifying a syncretistic mix of traditional and contemporary modes of performance, has been used in various forms and for various purposes since pre-colonial times. Quite a few reports and books have been written about theatre as a developmental phenomenon.[11] Some researchers hold doubts about the potential of applied theatre as an instrument for social reform,[12] while others tend to be overly optimistic about its capacity to instigate social changes.[13] A few studies have put community theatre in relation to AIDS, but they are either out of date[14] or limited in scope,[15] or lack epidemiological pertinence on a communal and interactive level.[16] The most probing texts on theatre and AIDS have been written in the form of reports by researchers and outreach workers such as Augustin Hatar (2001; 1998).

In the 1960s, the decade of independence in most African countries, the so-called travelling-theatre movements were deployed by university scholars aiming for cultural revitalization.[17] European-style 'well-made plays' toured and became a mobile vehicle geared towards rural audiences by university-based African artists. Like most development workers at the time, however, the plays did not pay a great deal of attention to local traditions or languages, let alone the gender issues that lurked behind societal predicaments.

In a second phase, theatre projects were brought closer to their target audiences. In 1974 the Laedza Batanani movement was launched in Botswana, marking the start of so-called Theatre for Development. This was also an academic project with built-in problems of involving local audiences in projects about communal challenges, but under the influence of Paulo Freire's 'pedagogy of the oppressed' project facilitators paid increasing attention to situational and political conditions.[18] About the same time, the Ahmadu Bello University in Zaira, Nigeria, took on similar projects, now also inspired by Augusto Boal's 'theatre of the oppressed'.[19] Artistic outreach workers dwelled amid villagers or urban squatters, composed skits and role-plays based on characters and scenarios as narrated by the locals, performed the result for them, and then invited the audience to alter the resolution of plots by way of simultaneous dramaturgy and post-performance discussions. The development of community theatre spread across Africa via international workshops and eventually led to a third phase of community theatre, elaborated in countries such as Lesotho, Zimbabwe, and Tanzania.[20] At this point most of the creative and edifying *modus operandi* were entrusted to the community subjects themselves, who participated directly in the planning and performing of the theatre. Community theatre went from being a social event to becoming a social process.

The third phase of community theatre coincides with the outbreak of the AIDS epidemic and yet it would take many years before the full potential of theatre projects would be employed in prevention programmes. When the first community-owned theatre projects were tried out in Tanzania in the 1980s, aid organizations such as WHO circulated Northern-style information and education on how the epidemic occurred, while religious organizations took care of the moral explanation of why it occurred (Iliffe 2006: 90). Not until the recognition of culture-specific communication in the 1990s would people's local knowledge and practices have a bearing on programmes dealing with their own predicaments.

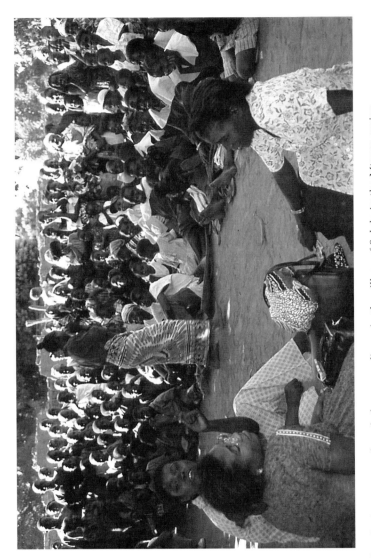

6  Three female characters perform before an audience in the village of Sululu in the Mtwara region
(Photo: Ola Johansson)

The ultimate objective of TFD and other HIV preventive schemes is to effectuate perlocutionary acts, or reciprocal performative speech acts, that not only express matters in a convincing way, but also persuade interlocutors to take subsequent action for their own and others' sake. Ironically, this objective does not seem attainable either by result-oriented performances or by didactic methods. I would not go so far as to say with Setel that preventive actions ought to be '*service* oriented rather than educational' (my emphasis), even if it is fair to assume that 'the impact of targeted interventions such as those promoting condom use may be very limited' and that the notion of 'behaviour change' is subject to manifold 'situational constraints' (Setel 1999: 245–6). It is clear that superimposed educational projects rarely reach the cultural profundity of behaviour change. AIDS has forced development workers to realize that cultural changes can only transpire through people's own initiatives and actions. Some CBT practitioners appreciated this epidemiological fact long before most aid workers and thus altered their interventions from being nomadic and ephemeral to be culture-specific and long-lasting.

In the 1980s so-called Theatre for Development (TFD) spread across sub-Saharan Africa through annual international workshops, which gradually improved its initial methods. The Laedza Batanani projects conceptualized and implemented its prototypical model, but also met with criticism on a number of counts. A few crucial elements had been overlooked, such as the use of local languages, indigenous performance traditions, and gender issues (Mlama 1991; Kerr 2002). Byam (1999) has also criticized the participatory deficiency in the early projects, especially in terms of Freire's idea of a gradual ownership of learning projects on behalf of poor and oppressed participators.[21] 'Conscientization', a key concept of Freire's, claims that liberating changes can only come to pass if subjects actively relate a critical awareness and dialogic praxis to the societal and historical conditions of their environment. Artistic development workers dwelt amid villagers or urban squatters, composed skits based on characters and scenarios narrated by the locals, and then performed them before the community for discussion and, ultimately, for action. However, the ethnographic pertinence of their performances needed further consideration, as the indirect depictions of local scenarios and participants took an unnecessary detour via academically informed rewritings instead of adhering directly to the culture-specific circumstances of the subjects of the narratives and performance practices. This led to the mentioned advanced phase of sustainable TFD which developed in countries like Lesotho (Mda 1993) and Tanzania

(Mlama 1991), which still typifies the crucial methodology of theatre projects on AIDS.

Freire's 'pedagogy of the oppressed' and Boal's 'forum theatre' had built-in methods and techniques for audience participation (Kerr 1995: 161 ff.) and made a big impact on TFD. Combined with African performance traditions, these practices created serious theatrical sites at the interface of artistic and social actions where interchangeable role-playing could take place (Feldhendler 1994). To work well, the process should not only be long-lasting, but also involve a considerable segment of the concerned community. One project in the Tanzanian region of Iringa went on for several years (Nyoni 1998). Another 18-month project in the Mwanza region, which will be the focus later in this chapter, focused on older men impregnating young women, 'which precipitated a crisis in the village leadership (because the story cut so close to the bone), leading to the dismissal of the chairman and secretary of the [...] drama core group' (Kerr 1995: 158).[22]

The Boalian 'shift of emphasis from theatre as a finished "product" to theatre as a continuous and alterable "process"' (Kerr 1995: 160) became crucial for TFD programmes. Ross Kidd writes that it is 'the drama-which-is-never-finished, constantly being restructured to extend the insights of the participants. Nothing is presented as a final statement: each new scene is questioned, challenged and probed for deeper meaning' (Kidd 1984b: 13). The critical turn from pre-encoded performative events to open participatory community processes eventually coincided with an analogous alteration in AIDS interventions. After a long period of largely unsuccessful prevention programmes in sub-Saharan Africa, a paradigm shift transpired in the late 1990s whereby self-reliant community development programmes displaced policy driven by experts and biomedical campaigns. Previous efforts had suffered from misconceptions about the complexity of the syndrome and thus the premises of countermeasures. Conveying information on behaviour change predicated on rational choice models from geopolitical contexts in the North brought about a fundamental distrust in target communities and had little effect as the epidemic spread to general populations. Ultimately the gap between expert knowledge and conventional behaviour compelled a change from information campaigns to action programmes that streamlined prevention projects with broader agendas on poverty alleviation, gender equity, and lifestyle negotiations (Kalipeni 2004: ch. 1; Campbell 2003; Holden 2003). And in order to cope with these challenges, it turned out to be unfeasible not to hand over more managerial responsibility to people within the communities.

Early on in the epidemic it was urgent to 'break the silence'. In her studies on Ugandan campaign theatre of the 1980s, Frank testifies that there were always two types of characters involved, those who knew about AIDS and those who did not (Frank 1995: 147). Almost like an extension of 'the old Mr. Wise and Mr. Foolish formula inherited from the colonial didactic theatre' (Kerr 1995: 160) or the Medieval morality plays of northern Europe, the campaign theatre against AIDS exemplified stock characteristics of 'human genus persona' (Frank 1995: 137), often targeting illiterate spectators who were themselves commonly depicted as promiscuous characters in need of pre-colonial moral values (ibid.: 90). The amateur actors were well aware of popular performance styles and local vernacular, but the topics were geared by international organizations with an:

> organizational framework to both acquire factual information through research as well as to pass the information on to the next element in the chain. In the workshops, however, the communication is made to appear symmetric. The artists are encouraged to ask questions and discuss the information conveyed to them by the workshop organizers. An asymmetric situation is thereby transferred into a symmetric one by giving the impression of arriving at conclusions in a joint effort.
>
> (ibid.: 100–1)

As a fastidious semiotician, Frank is actually in favour of the explicatory process whereby performances correct bad behaviour by reducing it to clear-cut personal traits (ibid.: 117). Even if the Ugandan campaign theatre was part of a national scheme that reduced incidence and prevalence rates, it now seems clear that such an instructive theatre misses various concerns of the epidemic. A cognate form of decontextualized performance can be found in the controlled workshops of process drama which functions as 'an affective engagement with the human dimensions of situations – an essential stage in any effort to encourage safe behaviour in a time of HIV/AIDS' (Simpson and Heap 2002: 94). This is suggested in opposition somehow to the public performance-based theatre for development. However, given the volatile sociality and poverty that underpin AIDS, drama in education and therapeutic workshops may work as discrete components in intervention schemes, but they are insufficient as outreach activity. As much as drama in education and therapeutic workshop models are worth for people under epidemic stress, there is still a need for performances with a wider communal appeal. Didactic theatre and workshop training primarily address behaviour change, but AIDS is about wider challenges of gendered and other ingrained culture-political lifestyle metamorphoses.

This is where the advanced forms of CBT meet the contemporary criteria of HIV prevention. Theatre mobilizes the most vulnerable risk groups, namely young people who represent more than half of the new infections in Africa. It activates these people in gender-balanced groups and allows them to express their experiences of AIDS through dialogues, which, in turn, invites spectatorial participation. Furthermore, CBT initiates a responsive space for local languages, habits, stories, humour, traits, issues – mimetic qualities which are integral in traditional rites and storytelling (Vansina 1985: 35), but which are also put in critical perspective by post-performance activities. For many young Africans, CBT offers a unique bottom-up approach to AIDS, especially if it is accommodated in community centres with connections to out-of-school youth. By entrusting them with this creative and edifying *modus operandi*, those most at risk become the subjects rather than objects of projects, which is exactly what is required in HIV prevention. An up to date implementation of effective community-theatre projects thus involves:

- social mobilization of local participants
- seminars lead by specialists on target issues
- training of dramatic skills lead by artistic facilitators
- 'community mapping' and other forms of situation analysis by virtue of the participants' local knowledge, preferably in gender and age specific groups
- script writing or agreement of scenes based on scenarios as analysed and propounded by the stratified groups
- practical rehearsals of the scenarios, involving traditional as well as contemporary performance styles
- presentations of performances between the groups and to the community
- post-performance discussions among actors and with present spectators
- follow-up programmes for the purpose of a sustainable forum – in the case of AIDS projects, preferably in cooperation with parents, schools, orphan groups, people living with HIV or AIDS, elders, health facilities, other non-governmental organizations, local gov-ernments, regional and national policy-makers.

The basic idea is to empower vulnerable groups by letting them suggest social changes through self-reliant action research and performance practices. They must ultimately take redressive action so that all concerned become involved, including those who cause the crisis and pose the risks. Needless to say, this does not always work out as planned. I will not go into detail about all the possible pitfalls, but a few examples will help show how performances can drive the experimental process to the limits of a fair local democracy and genuine prevention strategies.

When young people have a sanctioned space for licensed criticism, they arguably come closer to the driving forces of the epidemic than any other group. The main reason for this is that they share a window of opportunity to convey first-hand experiences before being cast in rigid gender roles, taboo inhibited speech behaviour, or defensive social rivalry. In most places, the epidemics are driven by sexual routines framed by blurred kinship regulations, prohibitive church directives, biased gender obligations, transactional agreements on sex and, not seldom, coerced sex. This is difficult to bring to light for older generations, particularly for men, due to their close association with prevailing sexual regimes (Foreman 1999). It is also difficult for foreign stakeholders due to the risk they run of stereotyping 'African sexuality and AIDS' (Arnfred 2004). Young people get involved because they usually have little to lose in terms of social status or political rank. They are by no means innocent with regard to sexual experiences or lifestyles, but they are the first ones to admit this while making attempts to work out negotiation skills across communal divides.

In Tanzania, like most other sub-Saharan countries, people gather when they hear the abiding traditional cue for meetings, that is, drumbeats and local dances (*ngoma*) in public hubs. The audience will likely enjoy choral songs (*nyimbo*) and perhaps also poems (*mashairi*) and acrobatics (*sarakasi*) before the theatre (*michezo ya kuigiza*) is announced. A leader may open the meeting by declaring the purpose of the occasion. There follows one or several performances that are well known to the audience, probably in the farcical vein of *vichekesho* or *vivunja mbavu*, perhaps a local form of satire (*tashtiti*; for more on specific forms of the in Tanzania, see Salhi 1998: 115–33), or a dialogic verse drama in the vein of *ngonjera* (Banham 2004: 242), which is every so often swapped for its contemporary stand-in, hip hop.

The format of these occasions resembles minor festivals. Once the open-ended performances lead to debate, however, the event turns toward a community meeting. This is also where it should become clear that the dramaturgical research on plot and action engages each and every spectator. For every laugh, sigh, snort, glare, shout, and comment there is a tacit answerability, which should be spelled out in discussions after the performances. These talks sometimes last longer than the shows and may involve local fundraising for widows and orphans. Various techniques and methods can set off a post-performance discussion, but two decisive questions generally trigger audience response: Is it true that what we have just seen is happening here among us? And, if so, what can we do about it?

The appreciation of the plays obviously hinges on more than local performance styles. Spectators identify with the familiarity of the plots, since both the actors and their behavioural patterns are usually well known in the local setting. This is a rough theatre with stories based on collective impressions and received ideas, with the sequencing of events agreed on spontaneously and always with plenty of room for improvisation. The liminal interface of the social and artistic is enacted with a negligible representational distance. It is as though particular strips of daily behaviour are grafted onto a shared arena and set into play at a slightly elevated tempo and heightened mood: the manner of speaking, the allusions, the jokes, the clothing, the props, the intrigues, the site and all the rest of the elements are, to say the least, lifelike – a situation where and when people play people, to paraphrase Mda (1993). There is indeed public agreement on the fictional frame, some actors are no doubt very talented, and there are lots of ingenious uses of Swahili proverbs and other witty colloquial expressions in the plays. At the end of the day, however, the familiar theatrical qualities are less significant than the open-ended performative effects, which entail a demand for a progressing social drama with the spectators. According to Mead (1964: 310) 'acting in the perspective of others' is a central principle in the organization of social life, a third-person perspective on the interpersonal qualities of identity. Such perspective conflates with the performative condition of enacting personal identities in CBT against AIDS, which may be a very sensitive undertaking in the presence of fellow villagers insofar as a young theatrical actor/social agent often performs quite realistic characterizations of scenarios that puts him or her in harms way by people that may very well be among the onlookers. Hence the aptness of a theatrical role distance, which may be coextensive with what may be called a social safety distance in the act of presenting one's self as other.

CBT appealed to and mobilized men and women aged between 15 and 24, who suddenly were wanted as aid workers in the most important projects in Africa. (When I meet youth groups, I usually tell them that they are involved with the most important job in the world and that I am visiting them to look, listen, and learn.) In their formative years, youths have a chance to alter traditional gender roles before being fashioned into normal citizens. This is a challenge as CBT taps into the local traditions of ritual, dance, poetic storytelling, and dialogue-based performances, at the same time as it combines these practices with contemporary modes of pedagogy and interactive theatre. At an initial stage of projects, groups are given funds at least for the pilot phase, including training by artistic facilitators and health-care personnel. Performance skills are then combined with analytical components like body and community mapping, a non-linguistic scrutiny of intimate and societal risk factors. Scenarios are discussed, preferably in gender-divided groups, before being rehearsed and performed in public meeting places. This is yet another advantage with community theatre as HIV prevention, namely that young people are able to break the silence on taboo-laden issues of sexuality, sickness, and death before and with audiences that have gradually become willing to ventilate their own private views in post-performance discussions. With the help of good drama instructors, the plays are followed by 'joker'-led

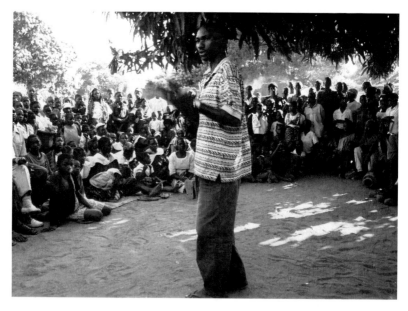

7   A Joker leads a post-performance discussion in the village of Sululu, Mtwara region
(Photo: Ola Johansson)

discussions as intricate as the plays themselves. With the help of good donors and local politicians, the projects may even be enhanced by sustainable follow-up programmes. This is all too rare, though, and an issue that I will resume towards the end of this chapter.

Hence the crucial activities of the social process are the performances which take place in public hubs such as marketplaces, schoolyards, or traditional meeting grounds. The events are commonly announced with hard beats on drums accompanied by whistles, horns or shouts, which, in turn, prompt a dance that community residents can take part in. I have seen about a hundred performances in rural African settings and, at almost every occasion, a decent number of spectators have turned up spontaneously. After the initial dances, the theme of the theatre is announced by the group leader. The mere word *ukimwi* (AIDS) may scare off a fraction of the crowd, but more often it sharpens the attention of the bystanders.[23] Short plays follow, resembling the comical verve in the tradition of Roman farce, *commedia dell'arte*, Molière and Dario Fo. The actions are based on improvisation influenced by local dialects, jokes and performance styles. When familiar characters are portrayed as villains in intrigues that everybody knows all too well, a peculiar alienation effect kicks in, which can be sensed like an uncanny echo after the roaring laughter. The conflicting emotions thus prompt the need for a communal meeting after the high-spirited events. The worth of an effective social mobilization of key epidemic risk groups, of a culture-specific employment of prevention practices, and of a persuasive appeal to the large numbers of local residents, made community theatre a serious factor in the fight against AIDS in Tanzania and several other African countries. There are good reasons to assume that it has had at least a contributing effect in three sub-Saharan areas with epidemic declines, namely Uganda and the Tanzanian regions of Kagera and Mbeya.[24]

After looking at, listening to, and learning from theatre groups in five African countries (although predominantly in Tanzania) over the past few years, I am convinced that community theatre potentially is the most efficient form of HIV prevention for young people. I am equally convinced that it is the least efficiently used form of HIV prevention. This has to do not only with money-driven non-governmental organizations, religiously myopic patrons, or corrupt local politicians, but also with the theatre practitioners and researchers themselves. To clarify the misuse of community theatre, I will now revisit a theatre project in Tanzania which took place in 1982 and 1983, at the time when an advanced mode of community-based theatre became established and when the first AIDS cases in the country were recorded.

## The reproductive misfortune of Zakia

The seminal 'Malya popular theatre project' got its name after a village in Mwanza region at the southern tip of Lake Victoria in Tanzania. It lasted for more than a year and epitomized what Penina Mlama calls the 'Tanzanian model' of popular theatre (Mlama 1991: esp. ch. 7). What made the project unique, according to Mlama, was that (1) community members participated in all stages, from the social mobilization to the resulting follow-up actions; (2) the elements of the projects emanated not from preconceived ideas, but from local modes of discourse and performance; and (3) it drew on an already established national movement of dance and theatre in Tanzania. (Mlama 1991: 95–6)

In her book *Culture and Development* (1991), Mlama opens with an intricate pan-African background to her work. Colonial history and Western capitalist contemporaneity are blamed for Africa's macropolitical problems, while European missionaries are liable for imposing a culture of silence through implementations of Christian doctrines onto the micro-political grassroots. These ideological contraventions have had repercussions in post-colonial times through autocratic African politics as well as top-down Western development programmes. In the same breath, however, Mlama celebrates the Chinese Cultural Revolution as an exemplary social mobilization and uprising, a propagandist delusion promoted by Tanzanian authorities in Mlama's formative years as an artist (Mlama 1991: 11, 24). In order to infuse an independent spirit in Tanzanians, Mlama puts faith in the ideological role of pre-colonial performances. This was a time when 'children [sat] by their grandmothers' feet' on 'moonlit nights' and got 'entertained and educated' by performances that served as 'a tool for instruction and transmission of knowledge, values and attitudes in initiation rites, marriage, death, religious rituals or public forums for behavioural appraisal, criticism and control' (Mlama 1991: 26–7). With a pseudo-Brechtian stance against entertainment, Mlama argues for an ideologically conscious theatre in schools and other public institutions and spheres, but comes to the realization that Tanzanian authorities were and are rather indifferent to theatre except as a mouthpiece for the ruling party (ibid.: 103).[25]

The Malya project took on the burning issue of schoolgirl pregnancies with triggering factors such as poverty, male-dominated schooling, political corruption, and the ensuing premature marriages, divorces, and prostitution.[26] It is interesting to reread Mlama's book in light of the AIDS epidemic for two reasons: first, because the first cases of AIDS-related deaths were recorded in Tanzania in the bordering Kagera region at the very time of Mlama's project (see Iliffe 2006: 23; Iliffe 1995: 223–4) and, second, because the project dramatized predicaments associated with social life in general, and gender in particular, which have later been dealt with as key epidemic risk factors. A performance that took place in 1982 about the schoolgirl Zakia, her friend Josephine, and the businessman Mandanganya is a telling case in point. He gives her presents and Zakia agrees to meet him. Zakia takes the presents home and sneaks out to go and meet the businessman. She returns to find that her mother has discovered the gifts. Zakia lies that the gifts belong to Josephine. Josephine comes to say hello to Zakia, but is reprimanded by Zakia's parents for corrupting Zakia. Then Josephine discovers that Zakia has taken away her suitor, so when the parents leave the two start fighting. The unemployed boys come to pacify them and offer to sell the gifts at the blackmarket. In the next scene, it is discovered that Zakia is pregnant but the businessman refuses to take responsibility. Josephine is also pregnant and is subjected to the same treatment by the businessman. Zakia's parents take Mandanganya to court, but he gets away with a very light sentence because he bribes the judge. The parents are infuriated and decide to seek justice at the village council. The play ended here because this became the entry point for the post-performance discussion with the audience on the issues raised (Mlama 1991: 118).

The discussion that followed this performance is still going on in Tanzania 25 years after the event, but now with even greater urgency as it directly involves life-threatening calamities and not 'only' enduring poverty, inequity, and social alienation. However, at the time of the Malya project epidemic issues were already embedded in the scenarios, albeit tacitly. In the section cited above, Mlama mentions the unemployed boys' dealing with goods on the blackmarket. This trade cut across the borders of Tanzania, Uganda, and Kenya following a war between the former two countries and a severe economic crisis for all three countries by the end of the 1970s. The blackmarket was operated by young males relying 'for food, drink and sexual services, on cafés, teashops, and bars, largely run by women' (Appleton 2000: 23). The grim historical irony is that Zakia, after becoming pregnant and being abandoned by Mandanganya, barred from her school (pregnant female pupils still get expelled without discretion), and probably driven away from home by her poor parents, quite likely ended up as a barmaid at a time when fishermen, truck drivers, and racketeers carried the looming and invisible epidemic across and around Lake Victoria.

The post-performance discussion in Malya also forestalled topical debates on AIDS by relating schoolgirl pregnancies to the paradoxical stance of, on the one hand, reproaching youth for their drinking habits, bad work morals, and disrespect for traditions that used to prohibit promiscuous lifestyles, and, on the other, acknowledging the failure of the community and parents to supervise the youth, let alone engage them in income-generating activities or other meaningful initiatives (Mlama 1991: 119–20). In the early stages of the project, parents thought that the girls, especially, would be corrupted by participating in the theatre. Furthermore, the village core group got into trouble with the African Inland Church, who protested against theatrical depictions counter to Christian conduct. The dispute was eventually toned down as the Church admitted that the performances reflected realistic rather than sinful scenarios. A much more serious critique arose when the misbehaviour of the village leadership itself was divulged. The village chairman was forced to resign after it became known that both he 'and the secretary had been responsible for several unwanted pregnancies in the village' (ibid: 125).

When it comes to epidemic risk factors, two phenomena were anticipated in the Malya performance. One was the 'sugar daddy' dilemma, that is, transactional sexual relations between young females and older men by means of cash or alluring gifts – for example, clothes, jewellery, holiday trips. This still poses a widespread risk in today's AIDS epidemic.[27] Another epidemic topic is corruption, a vast problem that not only conserves political pecking orders but also discriminates against people in terms of gender, class, and ethnicity. The combination of poverty, corruption and traditional gender ideologies reproduces disastrous conditions for young women and men as frequently today as when AIDS broke out.

Zakia reappears everywhere I go in Tanzania 25 years after the Malya project, from the Kagera region on Lake Victoria near the Ugandan and Rwandan border, to the Mtwara region deep down by the country's south-eastern border with Mozambique. Confirming statistical patterns, young women are regularly depicted as sexual objects, prostitutes, scapegoats, victims, and, quite literally, femme fatales. In Mangaka village (18 September 2003), I saw a performance about a businessman who seduces a secondary-school girl and convinces her to marry him. When she gets pregnant he immediately abandons her, with the outcome that she cannot go back to school or to her family and will have problems finding a new partner for future support. It is like a reincarnation of Zakia and her fate.

In Sululu village (11 September 2003), she staggers around drunk in a red dress on market day and hits unashamedly on men who happen to pass by on the *barabara* (main road). The performance is witnessed by a couple of hundred bystanders under a mango tree, while elders enjoy the action on a bench.

In Kenyana village (19 March 2004), she is coerced into having sex with the man who hired her as housemaid – and his two opium-smoking sons. At least half the village watches on, in company with politicians, religious leaders, and schoolchildren. The post-performance discussion lasts twice as long as the theatre performance and ends with an agreement to collect money for schoolchildren with surviving single parents (an analysis of this event is done in Chapter 4).

On the outskirts of Masasi town (17 July 2003), a bunch of spectators linger until dusk to see her put up resistance by punching her husband for leaving her and the children for days on end without enough money. At a marketplace in Bukoba town (30 August 2003), before a huge crowd of marketplace visitors, she gets deprived of all her property by her deceased husband's family and tries to hang herself. A neighbour saves her in the last second. A similar scenario occurs in Likokona village (19 September 2003), where she gets disinherited by her own brother, despite living in the matrilineal belt of southern Tanzania. She takes the case to court only to be double-crossed by a corrupt judge (for a more detailed account of this performance, see the end of Chapter 2). The story is frighteningly similar to Zakia's 20 years earlier.

Mlama's vision of an ideological pan-African theatre informed by the cultural regimes of traditional societies does not promise epidemic solutions, and almost certainly involves more risk than mitigation for young rural people. This will be a crucial theme in the chapter that follows. The pre-colonial order of kinship-regulated societies has waned almost everywhere in Africa by now and the social regularity and continuity of initiation rites involving tutored life skills for youth are, again, often particularly detrimental to young females. In order to go to the bottom of this predicament, the crux of preserved obsolete social regimes, generalized health models and HIV prevention schemes need to be clarified. In this chapter, the described gradual confluence of CBT and HIV prevention has revealed not how the two developments have come to be mutually stronger, but, paradoxically, how the similar lack of efficacy in the implementation and outcome of theatre projects today and almost thirty years ago indicates a fundamental resistance to change, both regarding HIV prevention and CBT. In order to probe deeper into the resistance to change, the next chapter will put certain types of CBT and ritual on a par and analyse the performative efficacy in the respective practices.

# 2
# The Performativity of Community-Based Theatre

The romantic notion of a pre-colonial Africa, where rites and ceremonies guided communities into harmonious lifestyles and infused a democratic spirit before democracy existed, needs to be put into slightly more realistic perspectives through an examination of the conditions and functions of ritual-*like* performances today. Along with further empirical case studies, there is a concept which advances the discussion of efficacy in Chapter 1 but also offers a means of typological comparison between theatre and ritual regimes, namely performativity. Performativity indicates (the study of) possibilities to instantiate notions and rules through intersubjective actions. Even if the concept of performativity is not always used in anthropological studies on ritual, the latter set of cultural practices is regularly ascribed functions and meanings that meet the criteria of performative acts. The dichotomy that will be thrashed out in this chapter cuts between ritual and theatre like a diachronic fault line between practices that may have conflated in function but always exemplified different meanings and values, at least for the ones assessing their roles in various cultures. Concisely, the dichotomy can be spelled out as a postulation: ritual does things with social relations while theatre merely comments on them (cf. Rappaport's stance below). This description sounds like a paraphrase of the definition of speech acts, the precursor of performativity, insofar as it inculcated the semantic capacity of words to do things rather than just describe things. The self-sufficient efficacy of ritual versus the more passive referentiality of theatre will be questioned in this chapter by means of, on the one hand, a discourse analysis of ritual theory and performance studies, and, on the other hand, examples that show that applied theatre against AIDS can be considered a ritual of affliction with greater efficacious potential than ritual regimes when it comes to counteracting contemporary epidemic crises.

To avoid cultural generalizations, it is best to situate the critique within a familiar typological field. Victor Turner, more than any other anthropologist, has allowed theatrical and ritual functions to be compared in the continuum that has come to be called performance studies, primarily in his book *From Ritual to Theatre: The Human Seriousness of Play* (1982). In order to understand his views on ritual efficacy, however, it is necessary to go back to his earlier research in Africa which, ironically, gave witness to the gradual disintegration of societies with ritual routines and functions, not least in regard to colonial interventions:

> In many parts of Zambia the ancient religious ideas and practices of the Africans are dying out through contact with the white man and his ways. Employment in the copper mines, on the railway, as domestic servants and shop assistants; the meeting and mingling of tribes in a nontribal environment; the long absence of men from their homes – all these factors have contributed to the breakdown of religions that stress the values of kinship ties, respect for the elders, and tribal unity. However, in the far northwest of the Territory, this process of religious disintegration is less rapid and complete; if one is patient, sympathetic, and lucky one may still observe there the dances and rituals of an older day.
>
> (Turner 1967: 2)

This passage from Turner's *The Forest of Symbols* bears witness to a transition period when Zambia, along with many other African countries, underwent its first years of emancipation from colonial rule, and thus faced the consequences of a complex cultural shift from traditional indigenous practices to modern intercultural customs. Relatively unharmed by British authority, the Ndembu had been able to retain their tribal unity, at least during the time that Turner conducted his famous fieldwork a good ten years earlier in what was then Northern Rhodesia (Turner 1957).[1] The anthropologist himself had the opportunity to observe continuous and still efficacious rites of affliction and life-crisis rituals; the latter type has subsequently become a paradigmatic example of anthropological discourse in line with Van Gennep's (1960) master trope, *rite de passage*. From a contemporary perspective, it is remarkable that precisely those geopolitical changes Turner associates with the waning conditions of tribal life today are perceived as key factors in the spread of HIV in Africa. Increasing demographic movements and cultural displacement have uprooted and fragmented local communities since the periods of slave trade and colonial strategies of labour division, but has of course accelerated in postcolonial times with modern transport systems, urbanization, and decentralized job opportunities (Iliffe 2006; Barnett and Whiteside 2002; Nugent 2007; more specifically on Tanzania, see Setel 1999). In the power vacuum that corresponds with this development, it is not always clear what function elder communities and traditional health practitioners retain. This is certainly the case in many places in Kagera and Mtwara, where contemporary party politics may have implemented civil rights and imposed restrictions in traditional practices (prohibiting, for instance, initiation rites from taking place during term-times of schooling), but where governmental laws and local rulings sometimes clash and conflict. In general, however, it seems clear that traditional authorities and practices are abating in social efficacy, leaving societies, not least young people, in a state of social limbo between vanishing traditions and premature policies.

The virus challenges the cultural dynamics of modernity like an ill spirit of old and yet no instituted or otherwise known form of policy or practice has been capable of tracing or pursuing its complex mutations in contemporary African societies. Stemming the onslaught of HIV/AIDS has been impeded by a number of social and authoritarian factors: an official reluctance to acknowledge its existence, an interpersonal hesitancy to speak about its risk factors, a difficulty in seeing its asymptomatic bodily condition, a widespread discrimination and stigmatization of the sick, a resistance among governmental and non-governmental organizations to coordinate prevention programmes, and, for more than a decade, a corporate aversion to allocate biomedical means to treat opportunistic diseases. The result has been a paralysis before the spread of the disease. Hence, the AIDS syndrome at once thrives on traditional life and expands through modern life. And yet, as long as no vaccine is in sight and the anti-retroviral drugs are too expensive or difficult to distribute on a sustainable basis, prevention work through social changes and behavioural counteractions are the only ways out of the maelstrom.

In this chapter I will argue that, in light of ritual traditions and discourses, community-based theatre not only invents new ways of acting out and then talking about hushed up and hidden aspects of the epidemic, but also represents a viable alternative to former ritual practices as well as to daily discourse. In fact, its most auspicious qualities probably lie in combining these formal and informal practices through social mobilization, group consolidation, and certain modes of performative actions.

## Topical uncertainties of traditional practices

When Turner compared theatre with ritual in his last book, *From Ritual to Theatre: The Human Seriousness of Play*, he contrasted the Ndembu rituals with Western theatre (Turner 1982: ch. 2). Rituals are heeded as the 'work of gods', obligating 'communal participation' in liminal passages of the whole society through crises, while the leisure habit of theatre pertains to 'liminoid genres' of industrial societies where 'great public stress is laid on the individual innovator' (ibid.: 43). This distinction would not be very useful in a comparison of ritual and African community theatre under the present circumstances, at least not in general terms. Ritual is, of course, still a sacred and consolidated practice as compared with the more temporal and eclectic theatre, but when it comes to preventive efforts in the AIDS crisis, it is far from certain which performative practices serve more efficient communal and redressive functions.

Turner somehow anticipates this situation, not by referring to African theatre in his later work, but by recognizing the breakdown of 'ancient religious ideas and practices' in a book like *The Forest of Symbols*. The best-known ritual in Turner's research is, of course, the Ndembu boys' initiation rite called *Mukanda*, which belongs to a class of puberty rites in various Bantu-speaking communities of sub-Saharan Africa. This category of life-crisis ritual is indeed still performed, although on a more syncretistic foundation in most places. If Turner's analyses of the Ndembu rituals hinge on the 'tribal unity' of their society, yielding a 'total system' for the anthropologist to 'work out' (Turner 1964: 21, 29), as opposed to the more or less 'rapid and complete' geopolitical changes affecting most other communities in 'the world's fast disappearing 'tribal' societies' (Turner 1982: 44), then his prime example of a life-crisis ritual may accurately be understood as a historical instance – perhaps even an 'extreme case' in a contemporary ritual typology (Gerholm 1988: 196) – rather than an exemplar of how cultural predicaments arise and are coped with in cognate African societies today.

In his introduction, excerpted above, Turner links external factors to the religious disintegration that leads indigenous people to 'nontribal' places.[2] Long absences from homes due to migrant male labour opportunities along busy routes in densely populated regions have given the spread of HIV alarming prevalence rates in nations such as Botswana,

South Africa, Zimbabwe, Swaziland, Lesotho, and indeed Zambia. In the 1980s it became clear that

> AIDS was characteristically a disease of modernity, apparently unaffected by the natural milieu but responsive to the man-made environment of the twentieth century. This was because it was mainly transmitted sexually, often in association with venereal diseases, and therefore correlated with towns, transport routes, and labour migration networks where sexual partners changed rapidly.
>
> (Iliffe 1995: 270)

Some commentators have thus proposed nostalgic ideas about going back to traditional forms of sex education and other life skills informed by tribal regulations (Iliffe 2002: 224; Roth Allen 2000: Eyoh 1986: 17). However, while particular ethnic regimes could possibly gain temporary control of local epidemic varieties, it is difficult, if not impossible, to generalize the long-term prospects of such a restoration on a large scale, and, moreover, to know how severe the civic backlash would be for particular social strata. A crucial argument against the traditionalists is that many communities not only face an unsettling external form of communicable syndrome, but that some of their traditional practices function as social vectors for the viral transmission. In discussions of HIV and AIDS, a variety of traditional customs have been criticized, such as the multiple use of bloodstained knives in circumcision rites, unreliable witchcraft, sexual cleansing of widows, and the gender-biased commands of sexual and marital conduct in rites of passage. The latter criticism has also been levelled, albeit not specifically relating to AIDS, against Van Gennep and Turner due to their sparse attention to girls' initiation rites, that is, in Turner's case, the Nkang'a as opposed to the Mukanda of the Ndembu (Bynum 1984; Lincoln 1991).[3]

It needs to be considered, however, that condemnations of traditional practices often mask power motives of political and/or religious establishments that seek to win people over to their own particular agendas. In the AIDS context, traditional doctors are ignored by Western medical practitioners as well as by their African associates, as well as denigrated by churches, and marginalized by governments who advocate progressive modernity. Dilger emphasizes, along with Gausset (2001), that decontextualized criticism against cultural practices 'is not only unethical but also counterproductive' as it risks 'alienating the target communities' (Dilger 2002: 2) in AIDS campaigns.

Moral-religious discourses and practices may build the foundation for blame, stigmatization, and exclusion – and often for further HIV infections. However, they may also be a path for maintaining the dignity of the sufferer and his or her family in coping with the strong stigma attached to HIV/AIDS. In addition, cultural conceptions of illness may offer hope of being healed to HIV-infected individuals, and they have also become a means for families and communities 'of pulling together local worlds that are increasingly in danger of falling apart' (Dilger 2001: 11).[4] Whether informative discussions take place in/as theatre or through other public forums, ritual elements are in fact almost always part of social gatherings and, in extension, prevention programmes. They serve as a means to gather people together with drum-based songs and dances, which everyone recognizes as a summons to a public meeting. Ritual elements generally function as parts of, rather than as the monolithic agency for, such assemblies, and thus figure as 'multivocal' and 'polysemic' symbols, although not 'dominant symbols' to speak with Turner (1964: 32–5). It has become increasingly clear that no particular kind of action can assuage or resolve the complex issues of the AIDS epidemic. Multi-sectoral approaches are necessary to meet the challenges of contemporary pluralist societies, just as multidisciplinary approaches are needed in research about culture-specific epidemics.

Ritual theorists such as Van Gennep and Eliade tended to overlook the critical gap between cosmic and societal factors when attributing all-inclusive cultural values to ritual. Thus a long-lasting disciplinary fissure was established between ritual phenomena and other modes of cultural performance. Grimes argues that imposed patterns of cultural orders and practices were 'treated as if they were discovered,' which gave way, in turn, to prescribed models functioning 'as if they were laws determining how rites should be structured' (Grimes 2000: 107). 'Rites of passage can seem perfectly magical,' he writes, 'but only if you keep your eyes and ears trained on what transpires center stage. Backstage, there often seethes a morass of spiritual stress and social conflict (ibid.: 11). In a similar manner Moore and Meyerhoff state that 'ritual is a declaration of form against indeterminacy, therefore indeterminacy is always present in the background of any analysis of ritual' (cf. Layiwola 2000: 118). The question here is not only how the identity of individuals is transformed, or mystically transfigured, by being guided through transcendental passages in initiation rites, but also how such metamorphoses conform to the conceptual means of access of onlooking visitors. Seen through the ideological screens of Clifford's ethnographic allegory, where fieldwork is recognized 'as a performance emplotted by powerful stories' (Clifford 1986: 98), one is lead to examine the secular stage to which novices return and upon which the ethnographer stands waiting, as it were, to interpret their stories. Bloch (1992: 6) considers this return, from separation to reintegration, to be a quite violent step that displays the political outcomes of religious action.

Viewed in a critical perspective, ritual studies are predicated on the same secular conditions as performance studies, just as ritual performances are set on the same societal stage and in relief against the same circumstantial setting as are theatrical performances. The significance of this shared scene of inquiry is not a disciplinary issue *per se*; in the AIDS epidemic, it is crucial that all performative actions are assessed by equally critical means. Before suggesting the merits of community-based theatre, something more needs to be said about the justifications of comparing theatre and ritual.

## The ritual function of speech acts

Rites of passage certainly represent a venerable case of how changes in one's personal status can be instantiated through communal events. Ritual does not merely show and tell, it makes things happen in the local and cosmic world. A comparable, yet somewhat more discreet, example of such changes is established in speech acts, or what John L. Austin (1962, 1979) first called explicit performatives. The constitutive utterance 'I do', enacting wedding ceremonies, is a case in point, and is analogous to the notion of rites of passage insofar as both cases deal with situations where people's official status is changed through the performance of certain ceremonies. However, Austin's speech act theory does not deal with ritual *per se*, but with the possibilities for speakers to perform various social functions with language in particular circumstances. This eventually gives way to implicit performatives where less ceremonial statements like, 'I'll see you tomorrow!' bring about a commitment by binding the interlocutors to an impending event.

To realize the social pertinence of implicit performatives, consider a speech act exercise in a recent school workshop in KwaZulu Natal, South Africa. The goal of the workshop was to promote the ability of female students to say no to casual sex through forum theatre techniques.[5] The speech act in question turns on the proposition, 'I'll see you at 7', uttered by the male student Sipho, to which the female student Hazel replies, 'Oh! No, Sipho, my father would kill me.' Nevertheless, Sipho manages to convince Hazel, and she eventually gets pregnant, a fact that rules out further schooling for female students in South Africa (as well as in many other African countries such as Tanzania). The point of the exercise, then, is to go back to the proposal and find out how to turn down sex for one's own reasons. However, the project title of the workshop (instructed by the local organization DramAidE) was 'Mobilizing Young Men to Care'. Thus being able to counter an implicit performative is still contingent on the assertive interlocutor's willingness to rethink his subjective turn of phrase into a negotiable action.

Hence, speech acts may be 'highly developed affairs' (Austin 1962: 32) or quite ordinary events where someone wants to influence, warn, or encourage someone else, or perhaps just wants to 'let off steam in this way or that' (Austin 1979: 234). Austin views language as a binding means of intersubjective knowledge and trust, made to be performed for various purposes on the basis of more or less established habits (doing philosophy is incidentally only one of those habits). Like Wittgenstein's language games, Austin's speech act theory presupposes a culture-historic 'stage-setting' (Wittgenstein 1996: § 257) for utterances to take effect, even if the spoken performances appear mostly on the commonplace stages of daily life. With this return of the everyday voice into philosophical discourse (Cavell 1994: ch. 2), performative utterances can be perceived as 'a rare verbal form' (Barthes 1977: 145) only if the ordinary is somehow excluded from philosophical inquiry. Something similar can be said about the way theatre has been disregarded in anthropological discourse, even if a performance theorist like Richard Schechner (1988: 2002) has attempted to prove otherwise.

Very roughly, then, the idea of speech acts indicates a common ground of the ordinary, theatrical, and ritual inasmuch as all three areas of routine are more or less contingently based on, and geared to, performative conditions in particular situations.[6] As with all conventional states of affairs, any form of use can be abused or used abusively. The credibility of performatives depends on factors such as who the utterer is, in whose interest he or she is speaking, where and when the speech acts take place, how it is done, and, not least, what possibilities addressees have to respond to, or act on, the appeals the speech acts addressed to them contains. All these factors, each of which has the potential to impair the political and ethical reliability of a speech act, pertain to the cross-disciplinary field of performativity, which in the wake of speech act theory has elaborated analyses of power-laden regimes nestling in bodily and discursive practices, not the least of which pertain to speech act situations (cf. Butler 1997).

Speech acts are highly relevant to discuss in African CBT, even if what will be argued in favour of such an application does not sit easily with some theorists of bordering disciplines. Theatre appears to have become stuck in a functional continuum between the stream of direct interactions of daily life and the repetitive, more closed structures of formal ritual. For anthropologists and sociologists respectively, theatre seems to have something in common with both fields and yet not enough of either to qualify as a genuine disciplinary example. On the one hand, a sociologist like Goffman makes a distinction between face-to-face interactions (Goffman 1974: 8, 133) in daily situations in opposition to theatrical events, a distinction which hinges on a highly generalized theatrical frame (ibid.: ch. 5). On the other hand, an anthropologist like Rappaport (1999) separates ritual from theatre on account of an equally rigid opposition based on a presupposition that has been summarized as follows: 'While theatre confines itself to saying things about social relationships, ritual also does things with them; and what it does is to reinforce or change them' (Green 1995: 923). In other words, ritual does things with social relations, just as speech acts do things with words, while theatre is merely capable of commenting on people's status and relations.[7] In an additional move away from both everyday situations and theatrical events, Rappaport claims a prominent status for rituals by using Austin's taxonomy:

> [I]f performatives are understood to be conventional acts achieving conventional effects then ritual is not simply performative, but meta-performative as well, for it not only brings conventional states of affairs into being, but may also establish the very conventions in terms of which those conventional effects are realized.
>
> (Rappaport 1999: 278–9)

Rappaport is right in saying that ritual establishes its own conventions for performative effects, but he is incorrect in suggesting that this also makes it meta-performative, for that would mean that it could control the need and effects of its actions. That is, of course, up to people to decide over time and in reciprocity with their current living conditions, given that they reside in a democracy. It is obvious that a performance cannot (re)establish its own action more than an explicit performative; to enunciate and concurrently enact the conventions of a speech act is the very idea of Austin's doctrine.[8]

Schechner agrees with Turner on the dichotomy of theatre as entertaining leisure versus ritual as efficacious action, even if he makes sure to add that '[n]o performance, however, is pure efficacy or pure entertainment' (2002: 622). '[I]n all entertainment there is some efficacy and in all ritual there is some theatre', Schechner states (1988: 138). Schechner is also in agreement with Rappaport's view that '[p]erformances of ritual regulate or even create economic, political and religious relations among people who are ambivalent about each other.' Rappaport is quoted as saying that 'ritual, particularly in the context of a ritual cycle, operates as a regulating mechanism in a system, or set of interlocking systems' (Rappaport 1968: 4, quoted in Schechner 2002: 620). There is no doubt about ritual ruling as long as it controls the conventions and state of affairs it enacts. Trouble arises, however, when traditional systems lose coherence and validity in major crises. Examples are colonial rule, times of warfare, demographic shifts leading to multicultural societies, or, when rites of affliction not only must cope with 'internal changes' (Turner 1982: 21) but with the very endurance of districts and regions as in the AIDS epidemic. Even Turner, who outlines in great detail the anti-structural order of creative processes in the subjunctive mood of communitas during the liminal phases of initiation ceremonies (Turner 1969), acknowledges that there are limits to what ritual can change. Innovations in ritual societies can take place in legal and customary spheres, 'but most frequently it occurs in interfaces and limina, then becomes legitimated in central sectors' (Turner 1982: 45). In reference to what Turner calls ritual of affliction, Lange compares the social function of the Ukala ritual dance as it has entered into the post-colonial context of nationalist interests:

> Ukala fits well with the type of rituals among the Ndembu which Turner labelled ritual of affliction. In its nationalized form, however, Ukala is no longer a ritual of affliction, as it does not relate to 'abnormalities' or conflicts in the society. It is performed at any random time by national or commercial troupes to entertain a (paying) audience, miming a hunting expedition and the women who come to collect the meat. When the commercial groups address conflicts of today's urban society, they do this through the performances of theatre plays, not by traditional dances.
>
> (Lange 1995: 145)

For many societies, AIDS has entailed a critical discontinuity, which in turn motivates a need for what may be called 'ritual change' (Bell 1997: ch. 7). Theatre, on the other hand, can also be efficacious according to Schechner. In a graph Schechner (1988: 122) shows how contemporary paratheatre, experimental performance, political theatre, and performative psychotherapies exemplifies performances of efficacy more than entertainment. In comparison with ritual, however, it is not entirely clear whether this notion of efficacy holds. In order to consider the idea of an efficacious theatre I believe a crucial means of assessment and comparison is found in the concept of performativity.

## The performativity of community-based theatre

Due to its junctions betwixt and between the sacred and the pro-fane, orality and the written word, theatre is, according to Ousmane Diakhaté, 'one of the cultural elements that best exemplifies Africa' (Rubin 1997: 17). As Nigerian playwright Ola Rotimi has put it, theatre is 'the best artistic medium for Africa because it is not alien in form' (Gilbert and Tompkins 1996: 8). Yet drama with a fictional plot and narrative closure is a relatively new mode of public performance on the continent. Up until the independent states adapted its forms for their own purposes, spoken theatre was perceived as a colonial habitus. In its 'Africanized' styles, theatre has been and still is used in combination with a number of traditional expressions containing many ritual con-nections. Dialogues between characters as well as between characters and spectators have been an integral part of traditional gatherings, as, for instance, at the indigenous community forum of *kgotla* in Botswana (Banham 2004: 292). Village meetings have been narrated by clan lead-ers and elders, while fictional dramatizations have been performed through ritual mimes and skits or by storytellers impersonating mythic characters. In a sense, then, Africa had theatre before 'theatre' was brought to Africa. Regardless of questions of typology, the reality is that theatre is a forum for popular struggle both in national freedom drives and as a shaper of public opinion in post-colonial circumstances.

CBT is commonly described as a set of varied performative practices predicated on communal initiatives free from any consensus or author-ity beyond popular participation. It is certainly not a substitute for ritual, but it may be considered as a complement to it in some places and an alternative to it in other places. This is because it copes with communal issues by identifying the immediate needs of local popula-tions prior to the hardening of public policy decisions. Theatre as a forum for redressive actions allows community members themselves to renegotiate the validity of policies and practices, even if this comes down to substituting new actions for traditional rituals.

When Theatre for Development (TFD) was first tried out in the 1970s, it was in the wake of historical influences as disparate as colonial propaganda theatre, the travelling theatre movements of some newly independent states, and Paulo Freire's 'pedagogy of the oppressed' (1970). The pioneering Laedza Batanani movement (Kerr 1995: ch. 8) in Botswana was well aware of which historical misconducts to eschew and which good practices to pursue when it facilitated projects with rural communities. As mentioned in the first chapter, the basic concept of TFD was established by the mobilization of local residents around public performances that would trigger audience discussion and lead to their active participation in site-specific resolutions of social and material predicaments. Kerr understands the start of the movement in light of a post-colonial aftermath, and calls the performances an

> 'induced' popular theatre in that they have often been created in cultures like that of Botswana and Zambia where the migrant labour system or rapid urbanization has eroded most 'organic' forms of indigenous popular theatre, creating a vacuum which popular theatre 'induced' by intellectuals has been able to fill.
>
> (Kerr 1995: 152)[9]

It is interesting to note that the geopolitical changes, which Turner relates to the breakdown of religious life, and which I, in turn, associated with contemporary epidemic patterns of AIDS, reappears here in the 1970s as a need for community theatre. Given waning indigenous traditions and weak civil societies of centralized post-colonial states, alternative local forums were required to raise awareness and encourage participation on governmental land reforms, youth unemployment, health problems, and so forth. These are, of course, immense developmental challenges and eventually the themes of the projects took on more manageable proportions suited to post-performance discussions and follow-up actions. Since then it has been common to view TFD as means for pragmatic solutions, a quite confident opinion that had to be reconsidered in the case of AIDS. Digging a latrine in a TFD project is one thing, changing family structures and social relations, as in long-lasting CBT processes, are quite different. Even to implement a seemingly simple procedure like using contraceptives against sexually transmitted infections, which motivated some of the early Laedza Batanani projects (Kerr 1995: 152), has proven to involve highly intricate cultural ordeals in HIV prevention programmes.

Due in part to local needs for cultural regeneration and in part to the complex challenges of AIDS, two different modes of applied theatre have been deployed concurrently in AIDS campaigns: the first may simply be described as *performance events*, characterized by one-time performances of visiting theatre troupes or by individual appeals for particular media, occasions, and audiences. The second kind may be called *community-based theatre processes* and is distinguished by long-lasting collective projects involving local participants in social change. It is especially the latter mode of theatre that will be argued for as an alternative to ritual in contemporary African communities. However, the first mode, that is, the performances of group or individual appeals to people at risk, have played and continues to play an important role in certain epidemiological circumstances, especially in areas that have not yet broken the silence on AIDS. In what follows, I will give a few examples of performative events which have served to inform, persuade, and warn people of the dangers of HIV and the sorrows of AIDS,[10] only to conclude by elaborating on the merits of community processes as a viable succession to former ritual and syncretistic performances.

Individual appeals are not necessarily bound to theatre events, but may be expressed in classrooms, town halls, in bus stands, on murals, and through various media. Hence they could be a lyrical depiction of private experiences, like Philly Lutaaya's 'Alone and Frightened', a song that broke the AIDS taboo on the radio and gave the affliction a human voice in 1989 when Uganda was at the epidemic's epicentre (Frank 1995: 152–5). Sadly, the artist died of AIDS-related diseases later the same year. Invocations like Lutaaya's are cases of performative speech acts offered in the first person and the present tense by an individual who is living through that of which he speaks, that is, someone who embodies the status of doing things with words.[11] Due to widespread stigmatization and discrimination, few African countries have had prominent people willing to reveal their positive status.[12] Still, there have been a few in South Africa, for example, the young boy Nkosi Johnson and the AIDS activist Zackie Achmat. Achmat refused to take anti-retroviral medicine until it became available in public hospitals in the autumn of 2003. However, there have also been reports of violence against individuals who have announced their positive status, such as the activist Gugu Dlamini who was stoned to death by a mob after World AIDS Day in December 1998. In contrast, Lutaaya's lyrical testimony was encouraged by the uncommonly open and tolerant attitude of President Museveni's government in Uganda.

More commanding pleas have been voiced with illocutionary force through belligerent metaphors by political leaders such as Nelson Mandela and Kenneth Kaunda,[13] both of whom have lost sons to AIDS. Ensuing the death of Kaunda's son, the Zambian president declared 'total war' on HIV/AIDS, claiming that it ought to be 'not a national

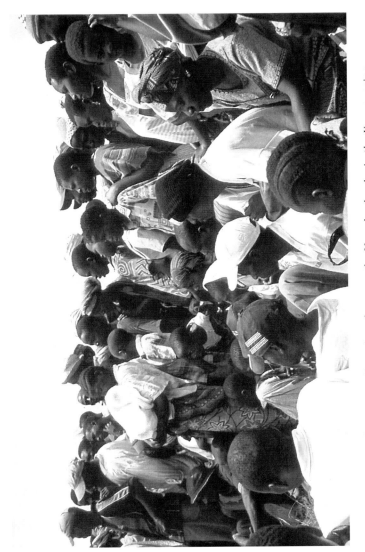

8 Audience at a community performance at Bunazi market near the Ugandan border in the Kagera region (Photo: Ola Johansson)

war that only appears in speeches at conferences and meetings but a war that becomes part and parcel of the life of this continent' (Sithole 2002; Nugent 2004: 358). The epidemic has indeed killed more people than all the wars combined on African soil in the twentieth century. If rhetorical artillery is fired too often and forcefully, however, there is a risk that it may avert attention from the already subdued voices and complex discourses among the most vulnerable social strata of the epidemic. One example of such complex and vulnerable discourse can be found in a performance I witnessed in the Tanzanian town of Kamachumu, where an orphan group performed the Omutoro, an aggressive warrior dance with spears that was once performed after battles for leaders in the old kingdoms of the Kagera region. Today the choral lyrics of the dance take on an emotional dimension when voiced by orphans in the local language Ruhaya, who cry out phrases like 'We have to kill AIDS!' Even if few of those who use belligerent metaphors spell out what kind of war is being waged, let alone who the enemies or allies may be, it somehow makes sense to see orphans piercing an imaginary enemy of old in the streets of Kamachumu.

President Kaunda's reference to conferences also makes sense, as they constitute a special performative site for valuable updates on research and policy making, but just as often come down to nothing but excessive spectacles of inert politics and detached science. In a number of counter-performances, action groups of HIV-positive people have interfered in meetings with demands for anti-retroviral drugs, as at the 2002 National AIDS Conference in Uganda (Wendo 2002). More recently, the 2004 World AIDS Conference in Bangkok, entitled 'Access for all', was recognized more for its disruptive protests than for its authoritative reports. A more subtle protest occurred at an international AIDS meeting in Dar es Salaam in 2002 by Frowin Paul Nyoni's play *Judges on Trial*. In line with traditional parables, the virus was invoked in this play as a supernatural entity that is constantly dissected and discussed by experts. In the end, the analytical paralysis of the scientists appears as a pathological side-effect of the syndrome itself. Like most pieces on AIDS, the performance gravitated towards a tragic end as the characters ponder whether anything can be done at all, although with an unexpected twist as the final question addressed directly to the experts in the auditorium was: 'But what should be done?' (Nyoni 2000).

An equally burning and open-ended performance took place at an AIDS conference at the University of Botswana in 2002, where Ghetto Artists staged a play by Vuyisele Otukile called *Salty Minds*. The performance begins with the rape of a young woman and her vain attempts to seek consolation from her father. Torn by generational conflicts, it is not until his daughter has died of AIDS that the old man regrets his conservative views in the face of his grandchild, who was spared at birth owing to a medicine (and a little luck) that prevents a mother-to-child transmission of the virus. Although the play reflected mainly male perspectives in critical scenes of attitude changes and decision-making, it did manage to cut across legal, religious, and cultural patterns through its daring depiction of risky behaviour in a country with a prevalence rate of almost 40 per cent HIV positive adults. The thematic accuracy of the drama was substantiated in the UNAIDS/WHO epidemic update, which reports that 'young women aged 15–24 years [...] are about three times more likely to be infected than young men of the same age' (UNAIDS/WHO 2004: 7). It is increasingly clear that these data are partially explained by sexual coercion or violence (ibid.: 7–18).

In countries with limited official information channels and media outlets, long-standing public events such as drama contests and cultural festivals have played important roles in raising HIV/AIDS awareness. A typical drama contest took place in 2003 at the Bahir Dar Cultural Centre in Ethiopia. The event brought together four so-called Anti-AIDS Clubs from as many Ethiopian cities to compete for a place in the finals on World AIDS Day. Four themes had been specified by the organizers of Save Your Generation and UNICEF: HIV prevention, stigma and discrimination, promotion of voluntary counselling and testing, and community care and support. Adopting a blend of comical skills from the Ethiopian tradition of *kinet*, each performance was given 20 minutes and a minimum of stage props. What struck me was how Ethiopian community theatre corresponded in plot, style, and characterization to performances at various youth centres elsewhere in Africa.[14] Ethiopian theatre does not derive from a ritual tradition as is the case in many other sub-Saharan countries (cf. Rubin 1997; Plastow 1996) and yet popular theatre becomes clearly recognizable across ethnic divides and national borders when young people relate its depictions to actual epidemic risk scenarios. One difficulty with Ethiopian theatre, however, is that it is tightly bound by authoritarian restrictions, which is detrimental to any theatre on AIDS. Restrictions are due to an entrenched alliance between the orthodox church and the government (arguably the most passive AIDS regime among the hardest hit countries of Africa). At the drama contest in Bahir Dar, sexuality and other taboos were conspicuously absent on stage. Despite a good act by a group from Debre Marcos that intertwined all of the optional themes, a troupe from Dessie came first with an unsuitably optimistic performance about a group of people who decide to take a test together and come out of the clinic HIV negative.

The political-religious fallacy is also a problem in Tanzania. In Mtwara region, where I conducted part of my fieldwork, it is not unusual too see Catholic public posters with explicit messages like, 'Don't Use Condoms!'. At a convention in Dar es Salaam in 2002, 70 representatives from a variety of religious faiths – not only Catholics but also Lutherans, Anglicans, and Muslims – made a joint public statement asserting that they will continue to discourage people from using condoms. This runs counter to Tanzania's national policy on AIDS, which emphasizes 'the overwhelming evidence about the efficacy and effectiveness of condoms' and the need for making them 'easily available and affordable' (*National Policy on HIV/AIDS*: sec. 5.10, 2001). Meanwhile, Tanzanian politicians are making statements that advise people to observe religious leaders. In September 2002, President Benjamin Mkapa gave a speech in Masasi in which he stressed that 'the disease could be avoided if people observe traditions, religious teachings and change behavior' (Mkapa in *The Guardian in Dar es Salaam*, 21 September 2002). It is quite understandable that politicians advocate religious organizations since the latter possess both the compassion and the medical facilities to care for people living with HIV/AIDS and for orphans. Their moral stance on HIV prevention is, however, the cause of misfortune, and this ought to be made perfectly clear when national AIDS programmes are designed and coordinated. Apart from the informative undertaking, then, an important task of community theatre is to clarify ambiguous official policies on HIV prevention.

To show and speak about the most precarious behaviour of the epidemic means to lay open closeted and intimate situations in the very act of underscoring their ramifications for a general tragedy. Theatre that enjoys freedom of speech and freedom of assembly often offers critical ways of perceiving intimate acts in performative stagings against multi-layered strata of historical and societal censorship. The presentation of sensitive topics – which has been and still is vital in areas with negligent governance, high rates of illiteracy, little or no access to impartial public opinion – by their very enunciation provides the conditions for what Austin calls illocutionary and perlocutionary effects on those who are ready to respond to the epidemic risk scenarios.

Despite the grim topics and motives, performances in community settings are regularly enlivened by eager audience comments and roaring laughter. One can always hear the spirited events from a distance. To a Northern spectator, they resemble comedies in the tradition of

Menander, Plautus, Molière, and Dario Fo, except for the mournful conclusions they engender when what appear to be stock characters run into economic and amorous trouble after challenging communally accepted ethics. Uncharacteristically for classical theatre, this leads them to existential crises, weakening bodily states and, ultimately, to scenes of death and funerals. Frank testifies that the plots of the so-called 'campaign theatre' of Uganda in the 1980s were almost always motivated by themes such as promiscuity, alcohol, and alienated women and men in urban settings. These issues indeed had an effect on the present onlookers, even if it is fair to assume that the reactions were ephemeral due to the cultural distance between audiences and the visiting troupes.

The travelling performances have promoted a shared sensibility for what lies behind abstract relations found in the extreme AIDS statistics, both for outside aid workers and local audiences. This sensibility is engendered by intimate love scenes wrapped up in burning political scenarios and the private experiences of profound anxiety and sorrow. Urgent issues of human and women's rights are embedded in local pockets of such intense depictions in ways that reports or papers seldom convey. It is a matter of ingenious inventions of action research – tender explorations in applied ethics.

Long-term CBT projects make use of both daily situations and ritual practices to entertain genuine speech act circumstances. Dialogues are taken from face-to-face encounters in daily life, yet with a role distance that permits critical depictions of public affairs and officials. Thus taboos can be opened up. At the same time an organized process is established, epitomizing site-specific features of particular communities not by means of a prescribed order, but rather by a participatory popular command in which self-reflective discussions develop through actors as well as spectators. CBT may not possess the ruling order of traditional ritual or engage the variable course of everyday life and yet this may not in fact be a disadvantage if the preventive prospects of intervening and redressing the afflictions of AIDS lies in negotiating *changing* living conditions. Both CBT and rites of passage set secrets in play, although in reverse ways. In initiation ceremonies, liminal phases turn social order upside down in a carnivalesque manner by including 'subversive and ludic (or playful) events' where 'people "play" with the elements of the familiar and defamiliarize them'. Here '[n]ovelty emerges from unprecedented combinations of familiar elements' (Turner 1982: 27), whereas CBT turns social order inside out by familiarizing taboos that have been defamiliarized in public. Hence the performativity of CBT, or, put differently, the coinciding effects of artistic innovations and social regulations, enact contentious negotiations on authoritative ruling and lifestyle options. The latter room for negotiations will prove to be the quality which is most difficult to establish and thus evaluate in the last chapter in regard to the implementation of long-term and comprehensive CBT processes.

All this is quite obvious in Masasi district today. On the one hand, traditional practices have gradually lost authoritative legitimacy in the multi-ethnic Masasi, but on the other hand, the very same practices can still be seen to play important roles in local affairs and are still practised in southern Tanzania more than any other part of the country (Mabala et al. 2002). In connection to celebrations, ceremonies, and other festivities performances, southern Tanzania offers most retained ritual dances in the country (Lange 2002). Few people would move into a purchased house without calling in a witchdoctor to bless the property from threats of, for example, jealous neighbours and relatives. There are still conflicts between local governmental branches and elder communities in the district about when initiation rites can and cannot take place. 'Traditionally jando used to be carried out at the onset of puberty, however nowadays parents often send children to the bush prior to enrolment in primary schools to avoid conflicts with the school system. The cutting of the foreskin is then done later during school holidays' (Görgen, 2002). The premature initiations are also considerably motivated by poverty, but in addition they have the detrimental subsidiary effect of very early sexual experiences among children and youth in Masasi.

Several people I have interviewed or had informal discussions with have confirmed that it is not uncommon with early sexual debuts, which increase the risk for sexually transmitted infections significantly. In connection to a project visit to Masasi, Mgunga Mwa Mwenyelwa, one of the most frequently consulted theatre facilitators by organizations like UNICEF, told me in an interview (Dar es Salaam, 7 August 2002) that an old woman in Masasi town had described the changes in initiation protocols for him. The woman had been initiated at the age of 13, but nowadays it often happens at the tender age of 8. Later on during the same visit, Mgunga got this confirmed when he started working with youth. One boy said that he had sexual experiences with about ten women at the age of 13. Mgunga also confirmed that elderly people in villages where the church is strong openly protested the divulgence of ritual secrets by the youth at theatrical events.

Moreover, widow inheritance is a traditional regulation which still exists and poses an epidemic risk in Masasi. In practice it means that a husband's brother takes over his wife when he dies. If the husband dies of AIDS-related infections, the latter will likely be passed on to his brother and, in effect, the brother's first wife, and so on. Furthermore, circumcisions are performed in the district in connection to initiations. In Masasi a matrilineal order is meant to protect women and their children from patriarchal control but this is also a regimen which is steadily waning. The latter system, along with some of the other above mentioned traditions, were exemplified in one of the most telling performances that I saw during my fieldworks in southern Tanzania.

The performance took place in the village of Likokona (19 September 2003) and divulged a notoriously vicious circle of epidemic risk factors relating to traditional regulations, topical policy-making, and youth, as well as women at risk. A widow has just endured 40 days of mourning, but still shows signs of distress. It turns out that her brother – the lawful guarantor in what was once a functioning matrilineal kinship system – has appropriated the inheritance to the detriment of his sister's welfare and her children's prospects for a decent education. The drama thus wanders between instances of legal and personal encounters. The widow knows that the law is on her side, but she is also well aware of the dilemma of taking legal action against a man with cash.

In an attempt to solve the conflict in person, the children are sent to their maternal uncle to explain their need for school fees and uniforms. The uncle maintains that their mother went to school for seven years to no avail, and that he will instead arrange marriages for the boy and the girl (Likokona is located in a Muslim part of Masasi district). The affair is then brought to a civil court, although the chances of winning the case comes down to who is bribing the judge with the most money. The brother offers the judge a half month's salary, while the destitute woman is not even familiar with the idiomatic jargon of approaching him with 'long sleeves'. What follows is a pig show where litigation is declared settled at a higher governmental level, and so the brother is cleared. Some senior people suspect corruption, but do not openly voice their protest. This taciturn attitude at the end of the performance is intended as an entry point to the post-performance discussion. But there never was a discussion in Likokona, most likely because the performance came too close to the communal predicament of corruption, or, put differently, to the impasse of being onlookers at an ongoing social drama that implicated political leaders.

Even if the performance in Likokona could be described in greater culture-specific detail, its basic course of events, nonetheless, points to a number of performative conditions of HIV-preventive theatre.

Performances do not have to spell out the issue of 'AIDS' for spectators to see that women and children are put in harm's way by being subject to unreliable governance. It is not just any kind of poverty that will force the mother into transactional sex and the children onto the streets, it is also a lack of legal and civil rights. The erratic order of things is, in turn, indicative of a disintegrated kinship system, negligent law practice, corrupt politics, and a defeatist stance towards education. Without trust in education (again, the leading proposal for discussions about AIDS among the focus groups in Masasi), the social status of young people is likely to perpetuate the status quo, which moreover sustains discriminatory gender relations.

Paradoxically, the vicious circle of the Likokona performance comes back to the theatre initiative as such, since the redressive possibility of CBT is to provoke a public response with a perlocutionary efficacy that can eventually lead to social change. In lack of a public discussion and official reaction, the double-bind with the man who buys his liberty with appropriated means, overrules his sister, and refuses schooling for the children, epitomizes a performative quandary of CBT, namely its difficulty in changing a social order despite, or rather owing to, its way of staging decisive problems in the very place and by virtue of the people at issue. If CBT goes far enough in its own undertaking it will enact its own subjugation – hence it indicates in this way both the possibilities and limits of HIV prevention for young people.

Much like Rappaport, Turner and Schechner, Hilda Kuper maintains that ritual is not theatre: 'It instructs through involvement, not entertainment. In ritual everyone must participate; no one can walk out or object to the subject. The participants are the audience. Though ritual is not designed as art, it is a sort of art – of masks, song, music and dance' (Kuper 1968: 90). Layiwola responds to Kuper by saying that 'it is difficult to draw the line between what constitutes a residuum of ritual, and what constitutes real-life theatre. [...] [T]he same elements "of masks, song, music and dance" which Kuper sees in ritual are the same for the total theatre event' (Layiwola 2000: 123). A 'total theatre event' in the age of AIDS should, to my mind, involve not only a form against indeterminacy and affliction but actually *involve* indeterminate and pathological factors in the challenge of given forms against a societal, ritual, and political backdrop. A total theatre brings out what Grimes mentioned as a 'morass of spiritual stress and social conflict' in the backstage of ritual performances. It is also worth mentioning a case of ritual theatre. In a community centre in the village of Mikangaula (17 September 2003) a rehearsal of a mime showed a male circumcision being carried out by an *ngariba* in the forest during an initiation (*jando*). One boy novice after another is forced down on the ground and cut without crying out load since that belongs to the test of endurance in the ritual. The brief performance was quite simple since it goes without saying that the use of one and the same knife for multiple operations poses an overwhelming infectious threat among the young boys. But the great achievement of the act is to show it at all in public. It is a text-book example of how a CBT performance can turn a social order inside out by familiarizing taboos that are otherwise defamiliarized in public.

Just as in the first chapter, the second chapter ends in a paradoxical vicious circle, an authoritative double bind. In the first chapter it was a matter of political unwillingness, while the second chapter indicates a cooperative reluctance on behalf of elder communities and, indeed, all too institutionalized academic scholars. Despite all the qualities that make CBT apt to offer an alternative to, or even a stand-in as, rites of affliction in the age of AIDS, it does not have the cultural or political support to reappear as such an alternative and to bring about real effects

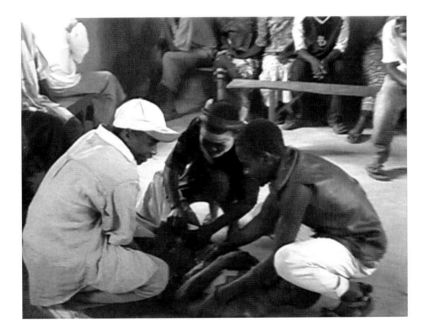

9   Rehearsal of a scene about circumcision in Mikangaula youth centre, Mtwara region
(Photo: Ola Johansson)

or changes. CBT thus risks being hollowly performative since, as Austin rightly points out, several crucial conventions need to be met and satisfied for speech acts and more complex performatives to take effect. Local performances may even work as HIV prevention by site-specific instantiations, or, put in an epidemiological lingo, as counteractive incidences, and yet fail to set off further ramifications due to its cultural and political seclusion. This is not due to a lack of autonomy or any other integral quality in CBT; at this point it is fair to assume rather that the very failure of CBT is indicative of a much more extensive failure when it comes to HIV prevention. It may even be reasonable to suppose that culturally motivated modes of HIV prevention inevitably will fail if a democratic and pertinent cultural form such as CBT fails to make a difference. And therefore the other side of CBT's failure may be considered a success, although in the bleak sense of demonstrating a rationale behind the failure of HIV prevention schemes in general (this reasoning will be elaborated in the last chapter). This is far from a futile task though. The capability of falsifying significant states of affairs or methodologies is an experimental achievement on a par with important breakthroughs in scholarly research and applied sciences.

In this chapter I have endeavoured to explain how the critical potential of CBT pertains to public opinion-making about initiation rites in southern Tanzania as regards, for instance, the careless use of sharp instruments in circumcision rituals, which was forcefully examined in a mime I saw in Mikangaula village, on the sexual tutoring of female initiates. On occasions when elderly people openly protest the disclosure of ritual secrets through theatre by young people, it is clear that CBT has the capacity of revealing conflicts that loom in the backstage world of ritual and how vital such revelations have become. However, more needs to be known about the backstage factors of post-ritual societies as well as the background factors of HIV prevention schemes in order to thoroughly assess and evaluate the potential of CBT to overcome the political and cultural resistance of its sites of performance. Hence instead of attempting to prove CBT's worth through yet another angle of approach toward CBT performances *per se*, the next chapter will go behind the public action and explore the stories behind the performances among performers as well as spectators. The next chapter will do this in reference to conducted focus group discussions and interviews.

# 3
# The Social Drama of Backstage Discourse and Performance

In the conclusion of Chapter 2 it was argued that CBT has the capacity to reveal conflicts that loom in the backstage world of ritual. The performative merits of CBT as HIV prevention has primarily to do with its task of bringing domestic or furtive behaviours into the broad daylight of public accountability. In order to investigate the correspondences and discrepancies between HIV prevention schemes, community performances, and potential outcomes, it is valuable to direct attention to discourses and practices between private and public events. In this chapter I will consider different kinds of discourses (group interviews, focus group discussions, and informal talks), which will eventually reach a point of an inverted theatrical and performative reality where confidential backstage talks allow for comparisons with official accounts of the epidemic and performances about the epidemic in the public sphere. As in the other chapters, this chapter is inductively piloted by an example of a community performance, which generates questions about the modal relation between the public and the private. A community group in north-western Tanzania, which could epitomize any manual with examples of best practices with regard to theatre as HIV prevention, turns out to be quite steered by the religious organization that backs their activities. Only because of a 'whistleblower' who was brave enough to share her misgivings about the condom policy of the Lutheran Church did I realize that even exemplary groups under the aegis of quite liberal faith-based organizations can be subject to ideological restrictions which ultimately infringe on the freedom of speech and liberty of association. The public-private fault-line manoeuvres the chapter into a couple of somewhat odd directions, namely a statistical analysis of the proposed topics of the focus group discussants I involved in my fieldwork in the regions of Mtwara and Kagera, and individual interviews and informal talks with audiences or ordinary people in the places where the theatre groups exist and operate. The backstage investigations point toward two significant findings; first, focus groups and individuals confirm the pertinence of the community performances when it comes to meeting the crucial challenges of the epidemic risk factors; second, the backstage discourse proves in no uncertain terms that the gender predicaments that have been suggested so far in fact can be considered to belong to the root causes behind the epidemic offensive.

## Part I

### Morbidity and commitment in Ilemera village

Ilemera is a village on the slopes of Lake Victoria in the Kagera region which I visited on several occasions during my research project. The village had a very well conducted community centre, with ambitions to obtain a set of best practices relating to home-based care programmes, social mobilization of village audiences, information meetings and theatre performances, quite methodical post-performance discussions, and bold follow-up schemes. State-of-the-art activities requires excellent leadership and in the case of Ilemera, the leaders were young and genuinely interested in putting up a communal front against the AIDS offensive. What follows is an account of Ilemera community centre and, in particular, one of its leaders who made a lasting impression on me on my visits to the village.

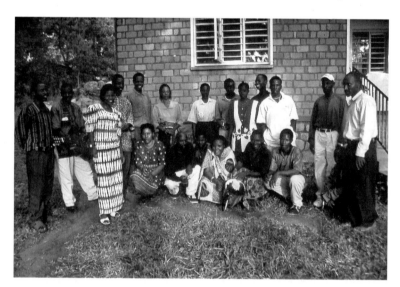

*10*   Personnel at the youth centre of Ilemera village, Kagera region
(Photo: Ola Johansson)

On my last visit (in 2006) D. (as I will call her in confidence) gave me a long, tender handshake and said that we probably will not see each other next year. 'Why?' I wondered. 'I'll be dead by then,' she replied and bursted out in laughter. 'God will have sent me an invitation to heaven.' I heard myself uttering something like, 'Oh, no!', along with a lame attempt to pitch her lenient mood, but my hesitant smile was pretty far from laughter. Shortly thereafter, I wished everyone at the community centre 'Kwa Herini!' But the farewell rang hollow inside my helmet as I and my colleague Stephen Ndibalema rolled down the hills of Ilemera on the motorbike.[1]

Usually we talked eagerly after our village visits along the potholed dirt roads along the lake, but this time there was not much to say. I had often asked my assistants, in Kagera as well as Mtwara, how close to the epidemic risks they thought the community youth were and they had always answered that they were at least as susceptible as every other young cohort. In spite of this awareness it was hard to accept that D., who at twenty something years was already a professional peer educator and action researcher, was in the grip of the syndrome. Certainly I noticed that she had slimmed a bit since my last visit a couple of years earlier, but it was as if her unselfish way of laying out the local context of AIDS, along with her enthusiastic appearance, made me look upon her as someone who could not possibly be dying. But that was the grim irony here: the ones who helped others to survive were often also busy surviving – and dying.

This meeting occurred at an exceptional time in the 25-year history of AIDS in Tanzania. Just a few years ago, around 2005, free anti-retroviral (ARV) drugs were allocated to selected hospitals in Kagera and other Tanzanian regions. Some people I met, a few of whom were friends from previous trips, were actually alive solely due to ARV therapies funded by organizations like the William J. Clinton Foundation.[2] There can be no doubt about the importance of medical campaigns at the present time. However, it is equally important to point out that medical interventions will not alleviate the spread of HIV, but rather mitigate the impact of AIDS for a certain number of people, at least as long as programmes are externally funded. For poor people in lack of a varied diet, the ARVs can also be a painful physical challenge. In a group interview (2 August 2006) with a People Living with HIV/AIDS (PLWHA) group in Kamachumu, a few miles north of Ilemera, a number of women claimed that they suffered so badly from the strong medicine on empty stomachs that the responsibility for their children ultimately kept them from quitting their life-saving therapy altogether. Such complications have brought ARV campaigns together with World Food Programme (WFP) interventions in some Tanzanian regions – although not in Kagera, which is a paradoxical region insofar as it generally has sufficient food supplies while also having the lowest per capita GDP in the country.[3] Even the best future scenario according to leading epidemiologists, however, reveals that less than one-third of AIDS sufferers will be reached by ARVs in the next ten years. This speaks volumes about the necessity of sustaining the development of HIV prevention work.

It is therefore important to justify why and how it is always necessary to involve social and cultural factors in any attempt to mitigate the epidemic – even if a cure could be produced and distributed. The reason for this is that the causal problems of AIDS existed before AIDS materialized and they would certainly remain if AIDS was eradicated instantly. No media or performance conveys this more acutely and accurately than community-based theatre, through its syncretistic, eclectic, and critical associations with ritual functions, communal meetings, vernacular storytelling, old genres of Tanzanian performance as well as new interactive and international theatrical and pedagogical methods and techniques.

In the performance I saw (12 March 2004) in Ilemera, the doctor in the local dispensary played the cameo role of a man who dies from AIDS-related diseases about five minutes into the action. This dramaturgical pattern is typical for theatre against AIDS in Kagera: people die at the outset of performances and the remainder turns into a struggle for surviving family members. Kagera is situated on the border with Uganda, where the first accumulated mortalities were recorded in Africa 1982–83. Here almost everybody has at least one family member who has passed away due to AIDS. In regions with less explosive epidemic experiences, such as Mtwara, characters usually pass away towards the end of performances. The latter 'tragical' dramaturgy, where the incidence and the ensuing diseases lead up to one or another kind of peripetia, lays emphasis on the preventive responses to AIDS, that is, how to discontinue the spread of HIV, whereas the former poetics of death and survival draws attention to the impact of AIDS, that is, how to cope with the suffering, care, and treatment of sick, widowed, or orphaned people.

So the performance in Ilemera starts with a man, depicted by the self-denying doctor, lying lifeless in a grove of pine trees under the vigil of his wife. Spectators from a nearby village sit on the ground close to the action. The tense but silent scene soon erupts in a shriek as the wife meets the inevitable fate and turns into a widow. In accordance with the local custom, a mourning period of 40 days ensues. After that something controversial happens, arguably as dreadful as being bereft of a husband. It starts with the arrival of the late husband's younger sister, who confiscates all possessions of the household and it ends with the father-in-law claiming the widow herself. The post-mortal property grabbing and wife inheritance are part of a traditional regimen in Kagera as well as other patrilineal parts of Africa.[4] AIDS widows do not just lose their spouses but also their belongings and belonging, that is, their material and economic assets, quite likely their health due to the risk of having contracted the virus from their diseased husbands, and their personal status since the other losses are tied in with a social stigma that makes it hard to meet a new man and thus an economic guarantor.

Gender wise, the story may, of course, also apply the other way around. In one of her early songs, Saida Karoli, the most celebrated contemporary musical artist in Kagera, sings about a woman who wakes up in the middle of the night and goes to a bar called 'Tisa Tisa' (also the title of the song). The husband, who is depicted as lazy and unable to satisfy her, is unaware of the nocturnal excursion. When she comes back, however, the husband wants to have sex and so he gets the virus that she has just acquired. He later dies and the woman goes to the capital Dar es Salaam and sells herself for money. She comes back beautiful and moneyed, but gossipmongers suspect that she has AIDS. The alluring wealth of the woman still makes men attracted to her and so they too get HIV. It all ends with the woman getting sick, along with everyone else. She dies and the rest will follow. The narrative of this song not only illustrates the contemporary epidemic impetus and distribution, but also previous twentieth-century STI epidemics in Kagera, especially concerning syphilis in the 1930s and 1950s.[5]

In the Ilemera performance, the confiscation sparks a reaction in the community that prompts the village chairman to summon a meeting using traditional drums. When gathered, the villagers are asked to help the widow and her children, which they do by donations of goats, maize, and money. It is not spelled out, but everyone knows about the vicious circle of the scenario: for a woman and mother the outcome of destitution is all too often prostitution, one of the leading causes of AIDS in Kagera. Prostitution should be understood in a very wide sense of the word, namely a transaction between a man and a woman, where one of them receives goods, money, food, or personal protection for sex. For abundant historical and political reasons transactional sex for poverty-stricken women ought to be understood as a means of survival rather than a moral or promiscuous act, as many faith-based organizations categorize it.[6] A woman explains what prostitution means in her village, Gabulanga:

> It happens in the village, mostly through alcohol. You don't feel shy; you meet a guy who makes suggestions and you go with him. The day after you realize you have had sex. It's a simple way of getting sex, pleasure, and some money. The bars are located in private houses [the sign is a pack of cigarettes outside the entrance; author's remark] and it is not a matter of much money, but you get dependent. It's an easy way of getting money and pleasure. [...] The man may offer her clothes, while her husband is away. She accepts a gift such as a *kanga* (dress) and that becomes a form of prostitution.
>
> (FGD in Bonazi, 20 March 2004)

It is remarkable to see that an epidemic risk behaviour such as transactional sex also can be perceived as a lifeline for impoverished women. When they get infected, however, fellow villagers usually get the news quickly which means that they need an escape plan. This also affects widows. The woman from Gabulanga continues:

> Prostitution also occurs when a woman knows that her husband died of AIDS. These women are lonely and accept any kind of gift from men. They know they will die, so they turn into prostitutes. They are still beautiful, but lethal.
>
> (ibid.)

What often happens with widows, D. makes clear in an interview two years after the performance (3 August 2006), is that they dip into an emotional and physical depression since they fear that they are going to die themselves. After a while they realize, with retained vigour and sexual desires, that they must find a new way of making a living.[7] At that critical juncture, many leave their communities, where people presume they are infected, and head for the economically wealthier islands in Lake Victoria. If they are not HIV-positive before reaching the islands, they run a great risk of becoming infected by the fishermen out there.[8] But the widows have reached a point where they have nothing left to lose, which is not to say that they are at a point of no return; after a long period in which infected people are asymptomatic, they eventually start weakening in opportunistic diseases and then usually return to their villages to die. They still have a year or two to live and may very well attract a few men before the fatal decline. This is the vicious epidemiological circle in and around Ilemera in the district of Muleba.[9]

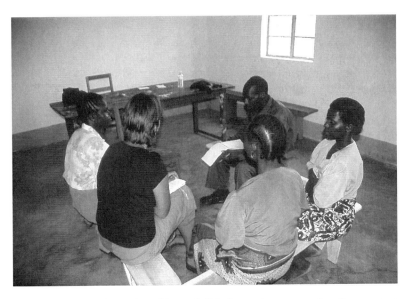

*11* Four women from the village of Gabulanga in an ongoing focus group discussion
(Photo: Ola Hohansson)

Donations can at best offer temporary aid for widows. In the village meeting depicted in the performance, a Kagera Zone AIDS Control Programme (KZACP) representative offers the woman a more sustainable solution, namely by proposing to resolve the conflict between her and her sister-in-law by mediation. In so doing the assets are eventually returned to the house of the deceased. Since KZACP also happens to be the organizers of the theatrical event, their involvement in the fiction makes the plot meta-theatrical – or, more precisely, performative. To at once depict and aspire to redress a cultural predicament that is widespread among the present spectators is to enact a perlocutionary speech act in the form of a promise that the audience is encouraged to act upon (cf. Chapter 2). Without the anticipation of a feasible audience reaction, applied social theatre, at least in this case, would merely represent an ideal scenario for the organizers and, in the words of Kerr, 'scapegoat the poor'.[10] In the interview with the Ilemera group it was pointed out that the same performance that we had just seen indeed prompted several women to come back to the community centre to seek assistance. They did not do so immediately, however, but tended to come the day after the performance rather than in direct connection to the post-performance discussions.

## The religious predicament

The meta-staging, nonetheless, made me suspicious about the group's sincerity and possible ulterior motives, not least because the main sponsor of KZACP is the Evangelical Lutheran Church of Tanzania (ELCT). Religious organizations have a systematic routine of promising people something with one hand while requiring them to pay back in faith with the other. Two things eventually relieved my scepticism; the first had to do with the course of action after the performance, the second with an intriguing renegotiation of Church policies on condom use, at least by informant D.

The post-performance discussion in Ilemera went beyond the typical performer-spectator exchanges conducted by the joker and 'spectactors' in forum theatre. The common follow-up questions were indeed posed – 'Are the events in the drama happening in your society?'; 'What did you learn from the performance?'; 'What can we do about these problems?' – but the 50–60 invited people, a significant part of a village, were divided into three groups that discussed the queries, presented the outcome of their talks, and then ventured into a shared dialogue that lasted longer than the performance itself. The occasion ended with a fundraising for widows and orphans in the audience's community – just as in the performance. This is something that takes place quite frequently in Africa, but that few people are aware of in the North. Before the meeting was closed, the leader of the theatre group offered the villagers a standing invitation to free counselling at the KZACP office with regard to the widow dilemma, a very audacious appeal considering the resource-consuming ordeal of such conflicts.

The second credible factor about the group had to do with their partial defiance of the mother organization's policies on condoms. In Tanzania all major religious branches are discouraging people from using condoms. This goes against the National Policy on HIV/AIDS,[11] which does not hinder the many politicians who give support to religiously authorized behaviour, that is, sexual abstinence until marriage and subsequent faithfulness. The 'C' in the ABC-model (Abstinence, Be Faithful, Use Condoms) is something church-goers talk about outside their houses of worship, as one man told me at a World Vision meeting in Kyaka on the Ugandan border.[12] His comment brought about an embarrassed laughter in the congregation that said much more than words.

When it comes to ideologically sensitive policy issues, attitudes often carry the significance of what is enunciated rather than the other way around. During my fieldworks I talked about AIDS on a bus with a nurse from a Catholic hospital in the south-eastern region of Mtwara. She held no religious qualms, but on the issue of condoms she said: 'Oh, that's a problem! I tell patients to use condoms when no one else can hear me.' In contrast to her commonsensical stance, most of her fellow believers prudently adhere to the papal commands of the Vatican. It is a matter of an attitudinal response to a principle, the opposite method, if you will, to conducting critical or scientifically valid studies. Should the Vatican lift its ban on condoms, people around the world would robotically do the same without any kind of reflective consideration and thus end the harm against countless people. As things are now, I can fully appreciate the passionate views of Reginald Mengi, former representative on the Tanzania Commission for AIDS (TACAIDS) and media tycoon, who criticized religious leaders' stance against condom use by associating it with the murder of believers who contracted AIDS from unprotected sex.[13]

The nurse on the bus worked close to a staunchly Catholic ward that happened to be one of my selected fieldwork sites, namely Mwena in Mtwara region. Experiences from that place have confirmed my suspicions of how religious dogma not only allow, but actively engage in doing harm.[14] My first visit (16 September 2003) coincided with – or perhaps prompted – a village meeting where I found a religious convener inciting a crowd of about a hundred people and at one point shouted: 'What do we think of condoms?' only to get the expected unanimous response: 'Bad!'. A little later I was invited to speak to the congregation. Diplomatically, I expressed a hope that all preventive and protective options are kept open and accessible for people without the financial means or social status necessary to make deliberate choices in critical situations.

The performance that followed by the youth group depicted a rather narrow scenario of HIV transmission. After having casual sex with boys in town, a young woman develops vaginal ulcers which turn out to be an opportunistic infection related to AIDS. The woman's parents first take her to a witch-doctor, but his treatment does not hinder her from getting terminally ill. By the time she is taken to St Benedict's Hospital in Ndanda (a Catholic infirmary near Mwena), it is too late and she dies. The unusually long death scene and its ensuing grief bore signs of scare tactics, again with emphasis on the preventive side of AIDS in Mtwara rather than the impact dimension in Kagera. The message comes across as saying that people will die if they have casual sex. The performance had an individual appeal with its focus on moral liability rather than a communal appeal with room for deliberation.

After the performance, I, as usual, expressed a wish to conduct confidential gender-divided focus group discussions with the women and men of the theatre group. For the first and only time in Tanzania, a community leader stepped in and hindered me and my colleague Margaret Malenga from holding talks.[15] Instead, we held a rather diluted general discussion in the presence of the apprehensive guardian of the faith. At dusk, when the latter man left the performance site, the remaining youth keenly asked Margaret and I about the reliability of condoms and other taboo laden issues. Again we kept a diplomatic tone and accentuated the need to keep all life-saving options open for as many as possible. I also informed them that HIV tests are free at the district hospital Mkomaindo in Masasi town a few miles away, as opposed to the Catholic St Benedict's Hospital in Ndanda where they charged 500 Tanzanian shillings for a visit and test. It is nothing less than a scandal that the young people of Mwena were kept in the dark about the free option at Mkomaindo hospital in Masasi.

Three years later (26 August 2006), I conducted random interviews with villagers in Mwena. A woman churning maize in her home, as well as people at a village pub serving home brewed alcohol, said that they had not seen anything by the theatre group for a long time and that the AIDS epidemic seemed to have gotten worse in Mwena and its environs. Of course I cannot ascertain a link between the local epidemic state and the tightly controlled theatre group, but it seems clear that the Catholic stronghold of Mwena impedes fully developed preventive measures against the epidemic through, for example, an iron grip around the young people's troupe. Statistically the villagers seem to be accurate: during my research project, Mtwara, the region with the lowest number of HIV testing in Tanzania, has surpassed the Kagera region in AIDS prevalence rates.

Back in Bukoba town in Kagera region, a Catholic priest told me that he advises against condom use and advocates abstinence by force: 'We have forbidden our members to have parties after six o'clock at night. If they disobey, we refuse to give them the sacrament in church.' (I remember thinking, 'Come on Father, who cares about reprisal if it comes down to having a good time and surviving a plague?' while pretending to be an objective researcher.) Notwithstanding the priest's rigid position, Bukoba town was full of stories in the summer of 2006 about late-night parties at the Catholic Church on Bunena Beach on Lake Victoria, with drinking clergymen enjoying watching people stumbling down to the lake for a quick one. At the break of dawn, the beach beneath the church is cleansed of condoms in waves of water – thank God!

Unlike the Catholics, the Lutherans and the Muslims are slightly less dogmatic when it comes to banning contraceptives. A theatre troupe from Bukoba, which I have seen and travelled with a number of times, regularly dramatize scenarios with condoms in their performances, despite relying on the support of the Lutheran Church. Coincidentally, the Ilemera group is supported by the same diocese. When I and Stephen Ndibalema addressed the question of condom use in our interview with the Ilemera group, D. told the other leaders present in the community centre, with a surreptitious but emphatic aside: 'It is very important to tell them about this!' She went on to say, without explicit backing from her colleagues, that 'one problem we have – and this is a big one! – is that our sponsor is limiting our ability to talk about and distribute condoms.' In the same breath she showed me a book circulated by a Lutheran publishing company that lays out the text on the ban of condoms which they are meant to obey. Stephen later says that D. is a typical Abanyaiyangiro, an outspoken person from southern Muleba district, as opposed to the more modest Bahamba of the northern part of the district.

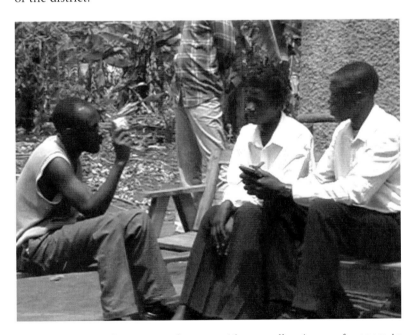

*12*  A young man discusses condom use with counsellors in a performance in Birabo, Kagera region
(Photo: Ola Johansson)

On the topic of condoms, a scene comes to mind from a performance in the village of Birabo (9 August 2006) near Ilemera. A man has an appointment with counsellors about whether to take an HIV test and the possible outcome of a positive (i.e., bad) result. The advice is that he should, then, make sure to eat well and avoid having sex. He asks if it is acceptable to have sex with condoms, waving a rubber in his right hand. A counsellor replies that condoms only have partial protection and that abstinence from sex is preferable. The man then concludes the conversation by making one of the most intriguing of social gestus I have seen in theatre against AIDS: the sign of the cross with the condom in his hand.

## The backstage performance of community-based theatre

It was mentioned earlier on how a performance initiated a post-performance discussion that generated a donation for widows and orphans and an organized undertaking to legally liaise with oppressed women caught up in unjust survival games. This does not only have to do with mitigating the impact of AIDS but also preventing the spread of HIV. The performance depicted the predicament of widowhood as a crucial symptom of the vicious epidemic circle related to patrilineal rule and its property confiscation, leading to destitution, which can, in effect, lead to prostitution, a leading cause in the dissemination of HIV in Kagera. In the post-performance discussion, the villagers testified that the vicious circle indeed exists in their community and that they would take measures to protect widows – even with the help of KZACP counsellors if necessary. Besides this, I conducted focus group discussions (FGDs) with the female and male members of the community centre, which verified the association of impoverishment and female prostitution. The FGDs also confirmed that the subsidizing church discourages them from using condoms. This is, of course, a serious discrepancy in the work by the community group in Ilemera. The latter is indeed one of the most advanced groups of action researchers I have come across in Africa, with an organization of outreach nurses, peer educators, coordinators, and counsellors. And yet the adverse stance against condoms can cancel out the possibilities to break the vicious circle of destitution/prostitution. In the group interview, however, there were not only mixed signals but also mixed opinions about the condom issue.

This is where informant D. comes into the picture, a dissident who was ready to speak out against contradictory principles and practices in favour of epidemiologically, ethically, and politically motivated actions – even in defiance of her financial and moral benefactor. It is highly likely that optimistic statistical data about declining incidence rates and prevalence trends encourage extension workers in communities to pursue what they consider to be efficient and true, in defiance of commands and dogmas. Invaluable informants such as D. make the 'backstage performances' of interviews as revealing as the theatrical events.[16]

Another informant who put his own leadership position at stake was a young man whom we interviewed in a community centre in Ijumbe (4 August 2006). He told us a story about the time when the governing political party Chama Cha Mapinduzi (CCM) suddenly discontinued their funding for the theatre group. The reason, he explained, while anxiously looking over his shoulder repeatedly through the glassless window frames to see that no one in the village could hear him, was that a member of the rival party Chama Cha Demokrasia na Maendeleo (CHADEMA) took on a leadership role in the community centre for a period of time. Democracy, even in one of Africa's most stable nations, is quite restricted at community level, certainly institutionally, although in particular in informal situations involving ordinary people's everyday life. The most serious ramification of party political interests in regard to CBT is that it comes between the assignment of HIV preventive tasks and its follow-up component. This is where politics and health stand against each other rather than rely on each other for the sake of public well-being.

Informant D. in Ilemera says that as a peer educator she has now abandoned choir singing and direct theatre that simply alerts people against the perils of AIDS. That is a very candid statement which most people in her position would not make since they constantly seek more funds for their projects. D., however, is predominantly interested in efficacy. As paradoxical as it may sound, abandoning theatre can be an achievement for state-of-the-art community-based theatre. The latter course of action is about a broad action research methodology applying a variety of tactics rather than about styles or aesthetics. CBT, as it has developed in Africa and other parts of the world, is about intervening in places by calling attention to certain crises, mobilizing action-prone groups of people, letting them identify ways through or out of their predicament by means of site-specific performative practices: local meeting forms, action research, lobbying, protests, seminars, home-based talks, therapeutic group activities, and so forth. Such practices can be more performative than theatrical, as it were, and do not necessarily take place in public, but in private or backstage performances. Hence the objective of contemporary CBT is not to play theatre to communities, but to get as close as possible to a community's own discourses, practices, and human resources according to one or another scheme of efficacy. That may entail kicking away one's own ladder when cultural divergences are surmounted, projects launched and the ownership of programmes are handed over to groups on a sub-village level, through open-ended peer education training so that they can learn by doing on an independent basis. This is also how I sense the fate of informant D.: she is seeking out others to whom she can hand over her own practical knowledge of living and dying.

## Part II

### The social drama of AIDS statistics

Statistics may seem to be hopelessly remote from performance analysis of CBT, but it is in fact an inevitable part of the understanding of AIDS and its counteractions. Needless to say, my research methods are primarily qualitative in the form of, for instance, performance studies, culture-historical studies, focus group discussions, and interviews.[17] However, the epidemiological dimension of quantitative data can be interpreted as a qualitative phenomenon if the focus is kept on people's attitude to, and use of, the information. It is largely due to statistics that previous notions about AIDS as a medical problem for particular risk groups were refuted; it was surveillance data that exposed AIDS as a generalized syndrome linking widespread societal causes and implications with living conditions for people in prime reproductive age groups, especially the young female strata and their statistical overrepresentation.[18] Some well-functioning community centres keep their own longitudinal statistical data for the work they apply. This pertains to the centre in Ilemera, where recent statistics collected by home-based care units in the ward indicate that women outnumber men in HIV/AIDS prevalence rates.[19]

In Tanzania more than half of all AIDS cases are unknown, not only to epidemiologists but to the affected people themselves and their friends and family.[20] Few people go for a test and many live with the virus unknowingly, but there are also a lot of healthy people who lead their lives in fear of already being infected. Countless households live under a constant state of uncertainty and insecurity, leading to a defeatist or even fatalist attitude about AIDS as a personal and familial health concern. People pick up 'statistical rumours' which may drastically exaggerate or understate current prevalence and incidence rates. It is interesting to compare different views of the epidemic in terms of what Giddens calls a 'double hermeneutic', that is, the practical and discursive levels of expert knowledge and public knowledge respectively (Giddens 1984: 374). A consequence of the double hermeneutic of epidemiological statistics is that something wrong can be true and something true can be nonsensical; if a rumour leads people to believe a certain thing about the epidemic, then it becomes true if the criterion of truth is how people act upon information; conversely, a piece of information about the epidemic that it is not possible to act upon, even if it is valuable as a health precaution, is meaningless in practical terms. In the first chapter, the latter flaw was criticized insofar as Western prevention models based on information did not apply to African circumstances, while they certainly had an effect in Europe and North America. In this chapter, the other side of the truth paradox is crucial and can be viewed against the double hermeneutics of expert versus local knowledge; when a rumour or another type of informal information takes precedence over factual knowledge, it begs another type of epidemiology than the conventional one, that is, an investigation which comes closer to people's own understanding rather than what they are supposed to understand through medical knowledge or cognitive schemes.

I have met many people who believe that half of their community is infected, or who think that traditional witchdoctors can heal affected persons, as well as people who doubt that AIDS exists at all. Most people live and protect themselves according to their social and economic ability; beyond that they appraise possibilities and risks to the best of their ability, which is based on informal local knowledge; if that knowledge, in the form of, for example, hearsay – is a misrepresentation of an epidemic reality then that misrepresentation becomes an epidemic factor, at least for those who share the stories. Rumours may, of course, also point to accurate epidemic trends. That is indeed the case in the Kagera region, which at one point was the hardest stricken place in the world along with nearby southern Uganda. Substantial declines in prevalence rates in the 1990s have been corroborated in recent research by Gideon Kwesigabo and this good news has apparently reached Ilemera and many other communities in the region.[21] When I asked about statistics, D. maintained that one survey accounted for a prevalence rate of 9 per cent in Muleba district, of which the better part belongs to the district's 18 islands. Kwesigabo reported a prevalence rate for the Muleba rural district of 4.3 per cent in 1999, again, with almost twice as many recorded infected females as males. Since then the district has unfortunately exhibited rising trends in HIV infections among young people and blood donors.[22] Statistics can indeed drain a lot of meaning from studies by its quantitative mode of appraisal, but can also give a lot of weight to 'non-figurative' phenomena such as preventable mortality, gender injustice, and experiential uncertainty.

## The social drama of focus group discussions

An alternative mode of discourse to the direct and public post-performance discussions and the semi-confidential interview with community group is the confidential focus group discussion (henceforth FGD). Group talks in general are interesting liminal (or liminoid) social events. In virtue of mutually fostered attitudes, feelings, and opinions in closely knit social groupings, talks about cultural issues can be more revelatory in workplaces or in cafés than in domestic settings or in structured face-to-face exchanges such as counselling, seminars, or ceremonial meetings. This is also why FGDs have become such a popular methodological tool for social scientists and health workers, as well as market and media researchers, not least when it comes to private or taboo matters. To create a comfortable situation for participants in FGDs with reference to AIDS, extraordinary arrangements may be required. Certainly in my case, a lot of consideration had to be devoted to the leadership role, especially as I inevitably appeared as a white male European in pursuit of sensitive information on sexual affairs in Africa. Whether I wanted it or not, I had to play an active role in front of a target audience who would either react with awkward silence or enact more constructive responses. This role-playing is done without a script insofar as FGDs are 'unstructured interviews with small groups of people who interact with each other and the group leader' on the basis of a 'topic/question list' (Bowling 2004: 394, 395). FGDs are also a discursive key to undisclosed taboo issues such as sexuality, sickness, and death. To restrict my own position in the sensitive space of dialogues, pauses, and silences, I opted for an arrangement by which the interviewees themselves decided what to talk about. This was actually decided before I found out that such a method already existed and had a designation, namely 'Question and answer method', as suggested by sociologist Ahlberg (1997). 'The method is deceptively simple', writes Judith Narrow (2003):

> [I]t involves asking informants to write down all the questions they would like to discuss about a particular topic. While answers might then be forthcoming from the group, the beauty of the method is that the agenda for the discussion (the questions) is set by the participants.[23]

As a cognate variant of this approach, I simply asked the informants of my groups to write down the three most important issues about AIDS for him/her in his/her community. For the illiterate participants, the questions were verbally formulated to my research assistants. Hence a triangulation of factors of equal or similar importance provided a continual persistent framework for my 20 FGDs: you (*wewe*), AIDS (*ukimwi*), and community (*maisha*). The suggested topics relating to the three factors were then presented as subjects for discussion for the groups (cf. Appendix 1).

The statistics of 20 FGDs, ten in Mtwara region and ten in Kagera region, will provide a framework of the rest of this chapter but have already been touched upon in the analysis of the Ilemera performance. Thematic associations will be made within this framework of data, if not directly in the form of statistical graphs then in various contexts that point to correlations and associations between the statistics, the themes of performances, and the various modes of 'backstage talks' which I have conducted along with my research assistants. Later in the chapter I will go into more qualitative issues, especially with reference to a case study from Mumbaka village in Mtwara. But the first charts specify overall categories of topics on behalf of young women and men in theatre groups in what they believe is the most important issues to discuss about HIV/AIDS for themselves under their respective living conditions.

The most common topic proposed for the FGDs was education (Figure 3.1). There is still a need to convey accurate information and education about HIV/AIDS and its preventative possibilities. This is a need that reproduces with new generations of sexually active people, which has come as a bitter revelation not only in Africa but also in the North, where a lack of attention to the epidemic has resulted in exponential doublings in incident rates in, for example, the United Kingdom. Another rationale behind the need is that awareness about AIDS implies an extraordinarily complex comprehension since the epidemic determinants are social, personal, political, sexual, and medical. What makes it even more difficult to bring clarity into this complex set of knowledge, ethics, and life skills is the fact that so many different kinds of information have been disseminated out of governmental agencies, non-governmental organizations, faith based organizations, schoolteachers, parents, peers, and so forth. There is still a lot of inaccurate information and rumours that distort the perception of the epidemic. This is so not only in Africa, of course, but all over the world,

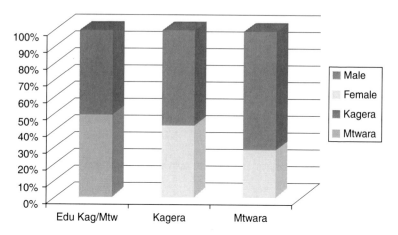

*Figure 3.1*   Mtwara and Kagera: education (category/topic)

which proves the point that awareness about AIDS requires a complex set of information and practical considerations.

Education should not be understood as a formal training in issues related to the epidemic, but rather as a wide-ranging umbrella term for knowledge about specific risks in relation to AIDS. To take an obvious example, the South African leaders Tabo Mbeki and Jacob Zuma are clearly well-educated men and yet ignorant when it comes to informed approaches to AIDS. The first doubted the connection between the HIV virus and the opportunistic diseases of AIDS, while the latter believed he could get rid of the HIV virus by having a shower after sex. These stances pertain to a particular male 'will to know' better than scientific research and can confidently be called uneducated in the sense of turning a blind eye to what is evident. Many cognate stances can be heard in talks with people in Africa and elsewhere in the world as regards sensitive AIDS topics (for examples, see the men's FGD in Mumbaka below).

Beside the fact that the ratio for the topic of education is almost identical in the respective regions (16 per cent for Kagera, 15 per cent for Mtwara), it is clear that the propositions from young men exceed those of young women. This is indicative of a typical gender pattern of the FGDs in general. Interests which claim outward going modes of communication and knowledge are typically propounded by young men, whereas considerations for more familial or intimate means of protection and care are typically expressed by young women. This gender

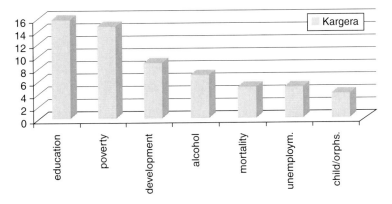

*Figure 3.2*   Kagera: most common topics (per cent)

dichotomy is less obvious in Kagera than Mtwara, probably because the groups in Kagera are much more familiar with informational campaigns by governmental and non-governmental organizations, whilst Masasi district merely accommodated a handful of organizations at the time of my fieldworks.

Figure 3.2 demonstrates which topics were most commonly proposed in the youth centres of Kagera region. Education has been mentioned as the most common topic for both regions. Also the second most common topic, namely poverty, is shared between the two regions. The third most common topic in Kagera is development (i.e., sustainable improvements in local or region industries and infrastructures), again probably due to the more established programmes and discourse on communal progress in the presence of aid organizations in the north-western corner of Tanzania, as opposed to the less recognized south-eastern part of the country. The fourth most suggested topic is alcohol/drug abuse in both regions. Mortality, that is, coping with the deadly characteristics and consequences of the syndrome, is a distinct topic for Kagera, where many more people have perished to AIDS. Unemployment, which is up among the most commonly suggested topics in both regions, is, of course, difficult, although meaningful, to separate from poverty. It is possible to hold a job and still consider oneself to be poor. Unemployment, especially for men, may also mean a lot of spare time spent in public houses and other social meeting grounds, which makes it align with issues of alcohol and drugs. The seventh most common topic in Kagera is a consideration about the impact on children and, in particular, orphans which brings me to

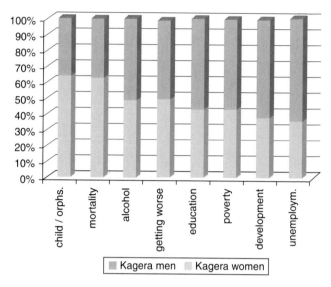

*Figure 3.3*   Kagera: most common topics among women vs. men

Figure 3.3. Considering the overall selection of topics, it is quite remarkable how dominant the impact issues are in Kagera compared to the preventive concerns. The near absence of the topic of condom use as one of the most crucial factors in the epidemic is ambivalent, though; everywhere we go and see performances and talk to people, the condom issue is raised in semi-clandestine ways since most places are tied to a religious sponsor. The issue looms in every discourse, but public ones and it seems quite clear that people are using condoms in sexual relations, regardless of religious commands. The relative absence of preventive considerations presents a thematic watershed between Kagera and Mtwara regions. This also shows in the dramaturgy of the community performances in the respective regions. In Mtwara it would probably not be possible to find a performance where a doctor enacts a dying man in the first five minutes of a performance. Even of the performance in Likokona (cf. end of Chapter 2) about the widow is almost identical in dramaturgical pattern to the one in Ilemera, the crucial issues seem to be about prevention and impact respectively, given the contextual factors of the performances. In Likokona, the need for preventive measures inculcates corruption, mismanaged inheritance procedures according to ethnic customs, and destitution as potential threats to the health and survival of the widow and her children. In Ilemera, the performance

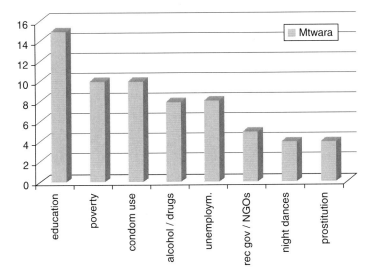

*Figure 3.4*   Mtwara: most common topics

appears to take issue with the unjust situation of a widow drifting away from a fair chance of getting reintegrated into society after the loss of her husband. The latter scenario not only jeopardizes the widow but the whole society, since widowhood is so commonplace in Kagera. Hence, while the storylines may be identical in performances in Kagera and Mtwara, the performative instantiation and the spectatorial perception differ according to the needs of the respective regions.

Figure 3.3 shows the same topics as Figure 3.2 above (with one addition, namely the opinion that the epidemic is getting worse, see comment below), but with a gender differentiation. It is interesting to see that young women are prioritizing private considerations of children and orphans as well as the mortal characteristics and consequences of AIDS more than official phenomena such as development and unemployment, which exemplifies men's priority. When it comes to alcohol and the opinion that the epidemic is getting worse (against the consensus of official statistics in Kagera over at least ten years) the distribution among men and women was almost even, whilst education and poverty were proposed more frequently among men. A similar clarity in gender divisive priorities could be noticed in Mtwara, although on the basis of partly different topics.

The most common topics in Mtwara (Figure 3.4) agree with the topics in Kagera, although with the exception of condom use, night dances,

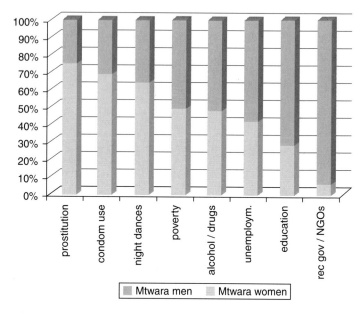

*Figure 3.5*   Mtwara: most common topics among women vs. men

and prostitution. Condom use may be considered an all too obvious precaution in Kagera, where the impact rather than prevention of HIV/ AIDS is most important at this stage in the epidemic. Night dances are more common in Mtwara due to a much more active tradition of ritual and ritual dances in the southern region (Lange 2002). Such nightly occasions are closely associated with unsafe sexual relations (cf. condom use) and transactional sex, commonly as a result of the consumption of alcohol and/or other drugs. The topic called 'rec gov/NGOs', that is, recommendations for government and NGOs is Mtwara's topic for what was called 'development' in Kagera. The relations of the progressive versus the more protective considerations make an interesting comparison between the regions.

Figure 3.5 shows in no uncertain terms how the most common topics suggested in Mtwara divide young women and men. Apart from the relatively evenly distributed focus on poverty and alcohol/drug use in the middle of the continuum, it is quite obvious that women are preoccupied with socio-economic links to sexuality in the form of prostitution, condom use, and nightly dances, rather than more external links to public sectors like the job market, education, and societal development. The pattern is indicative of a classical gender discrepancy

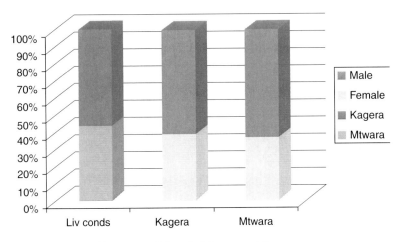

*Figure 3.6*   General living conditions in Mtwara and Kagera

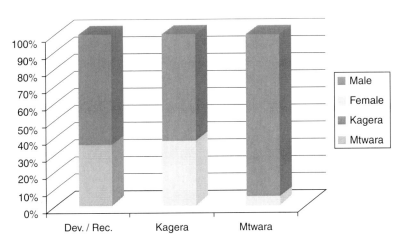

*Figure 3.7*   General living conditions in Mtwara and Kagera: development and recommendations

with domesticated and passive women versus mobile and forceful male roles. This deep and enduring predicament has proved to be a general pattern in line with a male-privileged division of labour and household economics in the most seriously AIDS stricken countries in Africa, such as Botswana, Swaziland, South Africa, and Zimbabwe.

Figures 3.6 and 3.7 show how frequent the broader category of 'general living conditions' were as topics for focus group discussions.

General living conditions signify a category of existing conditions and habits in society and domestic settings. Unemployment, which could very well be applied in the category of education and development, is here a condition rather than an activity; it could, of course, be seen as a risk factor that leads to casual sexual encounters by means of alcohol, which is yet another topic specified as a general living condition, but that could be seen as a direct link between of socio-sexual relations.

General living conditions are slightly more common topics in Kagera than Mtwara. The real discrepancy within this category of topics, however, has to do with gender preferences. It is more common for males to associate general living conditions as risk factors in the epidemic, especially in Mtwara where less than 30 per cent of the proposed topics came from women. The difference becomes quite apparent in Figure 3.7.

It is not only women in Mtwara who appear alienated from the topics of development and recommendations for authorities, but also women in Kagera, where less than one-third of the proposed topics of development were motivated by women. The topic of development (as well as education) denote societal conditions that the discussants wish to actively influence, improve, or change in order to gain control over HIV/AIDS (e.g., by recommendations to authorities and agencies).

Socio-sexual relations were mainly propounded by young women in Mtwara as relevant focus group topics (Figure 3.8). This is a practical category that indicates factors associated with the social environment

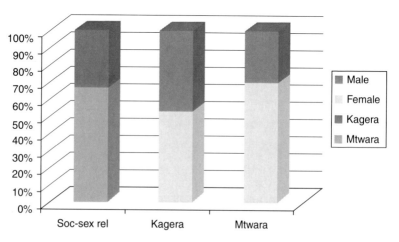

*Figure 3.8*   Socio-sexual relations in Mtwara and Kagera

and the interactive behaviours in sexual encounters. It is difficult, not to say impossible, to make firm distinctions between categories. Poverty, which can be identified as a general living condition, is 'hijacked' to contextualize the social and sexual vulnerability of women due to an often disproportionate poverty to the detriment of domesticated women with little influence over economic agreements in the household. There is consequently a need to blend the categories in order to make an interpretive analysis of the statistical data. Numbers, like words, are not innocent of context-specific meanings and values. To bring together categories of risk factors is a necessity for anyone who wishes to explore the potential to not only highlight states of affair, but also the possibility of showing their cultural and political contingency – that is, the possibility to change their conventional order. The next and final chart, Figure 3.9, is an attempt to reveal the gender predicaments behind the FGD topics by graphic means.

The graphs represent both women and female suggestions for FGD topics; rather than absolute numbers, however, here it is the different categories of topics that make up the gendered proportions. As has been suggested earlier, women seem to have put forth suggestions for the most important topics for FGDs by referring to existing living conditions, while men to a greater extent refer to eventual factors linked to

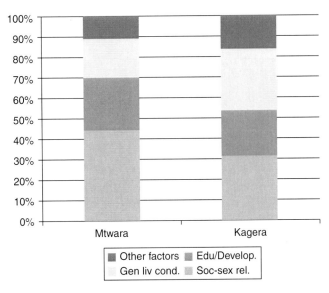

*Figure 3.9*   Gendered proportions of categories in Mtwara and Kagera

education and/or development. Thus a plausible interpretation from women's point of view is to align socio-sexual relations with poverty and other topics under 'general living conditions'. As a combined category this represents the main topics, that is, greater than both education and development, in Mtwara. In Kagera, however, topics relating to education and development are still greater than socio-sexual relations. ('Other factors' represent topics that are not directly associated with culturally integrated forms of HIV prevention, but which have more to do with the impact dimension of the epidemic, e.g., people living with HIV or AIDS, or topics which are so generalized that they do not fit specific categories.) The upshot indicates that a more advanced level of public opinion and developmental programmes probably brings the gender perspectives closer together, with the result of more consolidated groups and group efforts and objectives. Perhaps it is not, after all, a coincidence that Kagera region experienced a radical downturn in HIV incidence and prevalence rates during my fieldworks, while Mtwara region seemed to experience the opposite trend.

## Focus group discussions as action research

I will return to questions of statistical correspondences between performances and official data in the conclusion of this chapter, but before that it is necessary to get into close detail about the actual *modus operandi* of the FGDs. As indicated in the statistical trends above, one important arrangement was to conduct discussions in gender-divided groups and then conclude with joint discussions. A normal day in the field involved meeting a group in the morning, seeing their performances, eating lunch together (for the significance of the social climate of fieldwork, see Bowling 2004: 395), and then conducting the discussions. These are quite different types of activities in terms of time, space, publicity, and privacy. While the performances were public and the meals were more informal, the confidential talks needed to be held in 'found' spaces in public buildings or secluded open-air pockets. On rare occasions the talks were accommodated in intact rooms in community centres.

When it comes to the actual discussions, it was an ambition to be as unobtrusive as possible. This was a guideline for me but also for my assistants, who often, quite naturally, had the urge to approach individuals by way of ordinary interview techniques, or daily discourse. Despite the fact that I was often in need of translation, I decided that the only communication between my assistant(s) and myself was to be in written form between us once the topics were suggested and talks transpired.

It was quite clear that a reformulated query or a follow-up question after a silence of several seconds could spoil an imminent narrative or unravelling dialogue. On several occasions a lengthy pause led into quite divulging stories that in effect unfolded energizing discussions. The key to revelatory FGDs thus came down to a quite finely tuned balance between personal discretion, communicative openness, and attentive patience. The rationale behind my decision to combine performance analysis and FGD is that the latter can stand in as a form of performance in its own right when the former falls short as communication about HIV preventive conditions or solutions. In what follows, I will give an example of this alignment from Mumbaka village in Mtwara region.

## Part III

### A lost performance in Mumbaka village

The performance in Mumbaka Youth Centre (21 July 2003), an uncompleted brick house with a corrugated roof like most other centres in Masasi district, has to be considered as a work-in-progress. Most of the shaky plot is obviously carried by the improvisational skills of the performers, while the rest is acted out by physical gestures and interactions in line with a preliminary draft. It revolves around three young men in a public drinking house, who alternates between boasting about their own drinking skills and talking about the risks of AIDS. Two antagonistic characters quickly crystallize – pedagogically dichotomized between the attitude of enjoying oneself and taking care of oneself – while a third character mostly listens. The cautious fellow has obviously done his homework on HIV guidance as he paraphrases the ABC model of abstinence, faithfulness, and condom use. Hence the brief discussion about drinking and sex ends in a consensus reminiscent of Horace's classical criteria of theatre itself: 'Mix pleasure and profit, and you are safe,' as Horace put it.

In the next scene, women join the men in the bar. The man who earlier boasted his drinking skills continues to do so as he comes onto the women. He also makes sure to let everyone know that he is loaded with cash. Within seconds he has picked up one of the women and soon leaves the place with her. After a jump in time, the next scene shows how he picks up a second woman in the bar. His friends insist that he must be careful and remind him about the epidemic, but he is by now too drunk to take advice. After yet another hiatus, he comes back to pick up a third woman. She demands that they use a condom, but he pretends not to know what it is – and off they go.

After this there is a greater leap in time as we enter a scene where people prepare for a community meeting. To no one's surprise, the promiscuous man now shows signs of AIDS-related opportunistic infections. People gather, but a man voices a protest about attending yet another meeting that will lead to nothing. 'There is no water, the pipes are finished, this meeting is useless, for no one is doing anything anyway,' he claims. The protester then directs his attention against the sick man and says that he will leave the meeting if the infected man stays. Other people seem to take his side and so the meeting breaks up and is then postponed indefinitely. And with this open-ended situation, the performance also comes to an end.

The performance highlighted a few crucial culture-specific risk factors of the epidemic. Passing comments about failed irrigation and overt stigmatization allude to a relatively isolated agricultural ward with five villages on the arid slopes of the Makonde plateau. To get water up to those villages in the dry season requires a two-hour walk to the wells in Masasi town. The dry period inevitably also generated less employment since Mumbaka, like the rest of the district, is a primarily agricultural society. In July of 2003, people in this area had not seen rain for well over a year and in the periphery of the district along the border to Mozambique came reports of critical starvation. It is important to take such a geographical and societal backdrop into consideration when existential issues on disease are being dealt with in performances. Unemployment, poverty, and deficient food security are, needless to say, considered to be more pressing matters for healthy people than an epidemic with an incubation period of about ten years. The sick people showed symptoms, infections, and diseases which coincided with the local pathological environment, so under such vague epidemic conditions it is quite challenging to persuade people about the burning concerns of AIDS. A rhetorical question about poverty and HIV prevention that I heard repeatedly in Masasi was the following: 'What's more important to spend a hundred shillings on as a family provider: a bar of soap or three condoms?'

A more up front theme in the performance was the link between alcohol, money, and sex. This is a typical set of determinants for sexually transmitted infections not only in southern Tanzania, but also other areas of the country as well as internationally. If it is not about businessmen who pass by on the big district thoroughfare (*barabara*), it is about local village men – around or along smaller roads like the one passing through Mumbaka – who for one or another reason have managed to get some extra cash. An economic surplus is quite often used for either casual sexual affairs or more permanent extra-marital relationships. In the Mumbaka performance, the semi-official and semi-private regimen was merely hinted at, but was to be explained in greater detail in subsequent focus groups discussions, with the performers and villagers respectively.

As I and my research assistant Margaret Malenga made our way back up the stony dry road to Mumbaka village in September 2003, we had become increasingly wary of an additional thematic strand of the performance we had seen three months earlier, namely its gender partiality. Since July, we had accumulated a reflective hindsight of the Mumbaka performance by several visits to other youth centres and performances indicating a repetitive pattern of male-centred plots, male-defined problems, and male-driven resolutions. So as we divided the youth into one female and one male group for discussions, I did not expect a very vibrant talk with the women. On this occasion, however, I would learn a lot about the use and conduct of focus group discussions.

Since it was a Saturday (13 September 2003), we managed to find a vacant classroom in a nearby school. The four school benches that we put together for the talk made us sit in a square while an ideal option for a FGD would have been a circle. We were in the company of shy young women. When I now replay the micro-cassette and hear us introduce the initial topic to the group, there is a reserved giggle in the group. Then there is a long silence. The topic hanging in the air is about prostitution (*umalaya*). In the presence of reserved groups, the tactics was either to begin with the topic suggested by most participants or with the least suggested topic as a more drastic icebreaker that would then pave the way for an increasingly open discussion about less charged topics. In Mumbaka, we sensed that the women appeared shy but that they were consolidated enough to crack a taboo laden opener proposed by a single participant. The topics were, again, suggested anonymously and the only thing we know about their context was which three topics had been proposed by which anonymous individuals. The one who mentioned prostitution as one of the most important issues related to AIDS for her in Mumbaka also mentioned alcohol and the multiple use of knives in circumcision rites as personal/epidemic/social factors. Among the other suggestions for discussion, three were about increased condom use, three were about infidelity, another three were about sharp instruments such as the knives used in circumcisions, two were about the need for improved education, two were about abuse of alcohol, while single suggestions were made about blood transfusions and prostitution.

After the lengthy silence on the topic of prostitution, just as the taciturn atmosphere threatened to spill over to discomfiture, one of the women began to talk about evening dances (*usiko ngoma*). People get drunk, she said, and men ask women to come with them into the bush to have sex, most often without condom. It happens that women are with three men per night. It is not always agreed in advance, but women expect to get paid. If they do not get paid, they may abandon one man for another.

*Pause.*

Another participant offers an example. A woman comes into a pombe place (an informal building or site in which home-brewed beer and liquor are served) and come upon a bunch of drunk men. The latter do not jump at the woman at once, so she starts to dance and teases them as she says that they do not know how to have sex. She offers them to go with her so that she can show them what real sex is about. Then she promises that the one who goes with her will not be able to leave her.

*Pause.*

So far we had heard that, and how, prostitution takes place, but not really why it was so. The two initial anecdotes are like mini-drafts for an eventual play, although with female lead characters. A third participant then comes into the discussion: 'A man can know that he is HIV positive but since he has money he can attract women, who accepts him due to their poverty. It is impossible to know when he gives you the disease. Lack of food leads us into this situation.'

Here the pronouns starts to shift from third to second to first person and so the narrators gradually merge with the depicted characters. This is a shift from description to performance – a performative move out of the diegetic distance, as it were. The next informant who offers an example of prostitution again assumes a third-person perspective, but now in a dialogic form with direct speech. We identify the narrative as a site-specific experience, which may or may not be directly personal. In other words, the discussion is entering the same register as theatre and as researchers we feel invited into an at once group-based and subjective sphere of discourse. This is what is said:

A woman walks along a road and is being wooed by a man. Right at that stretch of the road there are no houses, so she gets scared of being raped. She says to him: 'If you wish to talk to me you can do it in front of a house.' Luckily there were people coming from the opposite direction so she now asks what he wants. He says that he loves her. She gets confused and says: 'So you love me? All right, well, I'm a married woman.' 'Well,' he says, 'I'm a married man.' She goes on to say: 'I can't cheat on my husband with you; can you cheat on your wife?' He replies that he loves her despite that he is married and then asks if they can go into the bush, just for a brief while. 'No,' she says, 'I can't go into the bush with you, especially since you don't love me; if you had loved me you would have wanted to know more about me, as, for instance, whether I am married or not.'

The anecdote ends here, in an open conclusion, just like a public community performance. There was no post-anecdotal deliberation though, probably because the individuals of the group had heard of the incident or similar incidents before and because they also were aware of its implications. A series of further anecdotes were then generated within the group, which had to do with women who go to towns for the purpose of prostitution; the inadequate AIDS education in homes, schools, and churches; the sexual magnetism of HIV-positive widowers so long as they have money; the difficulty for women to make men wear condoms; the lack of HIV testing among the young people of Mumbaka ('We can talk about it, but no one would do it even if the machine was brought here – even if they were forced by police or military.'). Taken together the narratives gradually expose the initial accounts about prostitution – the dilemma for women to, on the one hand, sell their own bodies in order to, on the other hand, protect themselves and children economically. This health-economical double bind is like a simultaneous inward and outgoing gesture, which is impossible to manoeuvre for an individual. To use a theatrical analogy, there is no possibility for a person to interpret her role if that position forces her to protect her life in a life-threatening way. There simply is no directorial method for such character development in the art of living.

When we sat down and talked to the young men we noticed, like so many times since and after, a considerable change of tone and attitude. What is striking is the men's demanding and even challenging attitude to governmental and other organized responses to AIDS. The gender discrepancy is given away already at the stage of suggesting topics for FGDs. Here is a sample of some typical suggestions by women:

- Women should stop prostitution
- Abstain from sex

- Use condoms
- We should respect out marriages
- Abstain from excessive drinking
- Avoid trying to get everything from other people (clothes, presents, etc.)
- Do not share injections or needles
- Do not have sex with HIV/AIDS victims

If the suggestions are not disapproving risky routines and behaviours, they advocate actions that are defensive. As opposed to this passive stance, it is easy to sense more affirmative and assertive suggestions by the young men:

- The government should look for medicine to reduce the sexual drive for men and women.
- Condoms are not the solution. People cannot use condoms properly.
- After an HIV test at hospital, people should be notified about their status, and if found positive, the patient should explain it to his/her family, to get the family's assistance.
- If someone dies of AIDS, it should be announced in public.
- Reduce the disease by drama, poems, and songs.
- They should provide us with media like magazines, video tapes, and leaflets to distribute to the villages.
- Show sick people on video.
- Youth should get educated on HIV/AIDS.
- Youth should get help starting income0-generating activities to be self-reliant.
- Authorities should bring as many condoms as possible.
- Authorities should also bring anti-retroviral medicines.
- They should bring testing equipment. There should also be a dispensary with a focus on HIV/AIDS.

Needless to say, the confident ethos behind these suggestions has not so much to do with personal qualities as a male licence to develop a critical stance to the social and political order of their living environment. Even where acknowledged risk factors reveal a defeatist or even fatalistic attitude, the assertive mode of opinion-making divulges a certain command of social critique and change. This implied command indicates, in turn, a more advanced stage for men than women along the Freirian continuum of conscientization and self-reflective praxis. It should be pointed out, however, that young men who have acquired life skills for a more self-assertive life face a discriminatory crisis cognate to the gender predicament for women, although in a generational sense in relation to adults and elder people. This will become quite clear in the light of the audience's FGDs below.

The discussion in the male group authenticated the assertive stance and affirmative mode indicated in the suggested FGD topics. 'Partners are not faithful and take risks without condoms. When boys want women, they don't just want to look at them but have sex with them right away. After sex many men abandon women. But the disease may already have spread – you may have contracted HIV.' Here it is more difficult to figure out the relation between the first and third person, but there is no doubt about the men's willingness to stand in for other men in the community, even if it should involve themselves. The men did not talk about prostitution, but another form of transaction that is just as detrimental to young women, namely the culture-historical phenomenon of bride price. In the relatively de-tribalized demographies of Masasi district, there are still evident remnants of traditional regimens which affect people in decisive passages of life, although in less institutional ways than before. Today a man can simply send a friend to the parents of a young woman and propose a marriage with their daughter by handing over 5000 Tanzanian shillings (approximately US $5) in an envelope. The parents seldom turn down such proposals, according to the discussion group, but the money is non-refundable if the young woman should refuse the marriage.

A related and quite astonishing subject had to do with initiation rites. The male and female initiations (*jando* and *unyago* respectively) used to take place around the adolescent age of 13, that is, on the limen to young adulthood. Today, due to waning traditions and especially in times of extreme poverty – such as the drought in 2002–04 in Masasi and other parts of eastern and southern Africa – families cannot afford to keep children in their homes and therefore send them to initiations at ages as low as seven or eight. There are at least two directly hazardous epidemic risk scenarios implicated in such circumstances. First of all, these children may be infected with HIV from birth without showing any signs of disease and consequently spread the virus if, for example, one knife is applied on several novices in circumcision ceremonies. (The irony is that male circumcision has been promoted as a major factor in reducing HIV in the last few years in sub-Saharan Africa.) The other risk is associated with sexual tutoring during confidential stages of the ritual. What is well known, however, is that the sexual instructions received by novices differ considerably between boys and girls. For young males in ritual communitas, sex is often characterized as a pursuit of manhood that should be conquered, while the narrative and physical instructions for young females more often takes place in a domestic setting that contextualizes a culture of subjugation related to the husband's needs. As a result, youth in Masasi district tend to have sexual relations at a very early age, which leads to a range of typical risk scenarios: reinforced gender roles, unprotected sex, untreated sexually transmitted infections, early pregnancies resulting in disrupted schooling for women, and so forth.

There is no doubt that the FGDs validated the thematic and epidemic pertinence of the rehearsal that we had witnessed three months earlier. A culture of poverty, alcohol and casual sexual relations impelled by money seem to lie at the centre of the epidemic in Mumbaka. A few questions remain to be answered, however, before a clear picture is established about the local determinants and the ways they can be counteracted. Why, for instance, were there no women in the leading roles of the play? Considering their ability to overcome their shyness in FGD, it should be possible for them to carry a public performance of theatre on the crucial risk factors of AIDS. And why was prostitution, or transactional sex, not a more prominent theme in the performance? As usual, it is also possible to question why gender inequity was not addressed more explicitly. What about the related dilemma of being a young person in a highly patriarchal and elder-oriented society? These questions all beg answers from the adult spectators who may sit on the culture-historical truths of the mentioned queries.

Three years after the rehearsal in the youth centre, I went back to revisit the Mumbaka group and to conduct FGDs with spectators after a new performance (23 August 2006). This was not to be. It turned out to be impossible to meet the group, despite intense attempts through discussions with the youth centre leader. The latter person was found in a newly established NGO, called Masayoden, which comprised the previous youth centres in the 32 wards of Masasi and Mangaka districts. The interest for specific theatre or HIV prevention projects in the new NGO seemed low; instead events and schemes had become centralized to a head office in Masasi town where rather more indiscriminate income-generating activities were planned for the villages and sub-villages.

The first thing we noticed when we arrived to Mumbaka was that the youth centre building was still incomplete. The UNICEF led project that provided walls and roofs for the youth centres had obviously come to a construction standstill at the pilot stage. We took a walk through the village with a faint hope of meeting a member of the centre who could tell us more about the fate of its theatre group. No one was to be found. So we walked back toward the main road and managed to recruit two focus groups for discussions on the same topic as we had done with the youth in 2003: 'Write down the three most important issues about AIDS for you in Mumbaka'. The men were selected from a group of people sitting under a tree in the midday heat, who appeared to belong to the same work force. The women were to be selected by a female volunteer during our discussion with the men.

The six men proposed to talk about three topics more than any other: alcohol, unemployment, and poverty. Prostitution, night dances, and unprotected sex were also mentioned although as singular suggestions. We started by asking what the group had to say about the link between AIDS and poverty/unemployment. The discussion directly took a turn, however, by the following opening line: 'Men don't know where to get jobs, so some become alcoholics. Bad behaviour follows.' Without delay the cue was taken up by a young man, who literally identified himself with the subject: 'I'm a drunk. After I get drunk I want any kind of woman that comes by. The brain forces me to it. I take any woman and don't remember it the day after. But in the morning I realize what I have done: I have had sex without a condom and slept with a woman I can't even remember.' Throughout this comment, which set the tone for the rest of the discussion, the other men laughed flat out several times. This is one of the best reactions a FGD can experience since a shared expression at once unifies a group and encourages follow-up comments with similar intended effects, even if it should be in another pitch and mood. That kind of remark came from an elder man: 'We drunkards are the problem, because when we get drunk we don't distinguish people; as long as it is woman we'll seduce her. And that's why the epidemic is so big: alcohol.'

At this point the discussion went from first-person speech to a collective 'we'. This is, once again, a theatrical mode in which depicted exemplifications and dialogues can enact the discourse in the form of direct or indirect experiences of cases against a communal backdrop: 'When you take alcohol,' another participant explained, 'your mind changes, your brain becomes wild and does anything. Any woman should be seduced. When you get drunk, the desire is high, but without alcohol you are a normal person.' In other words, the effect of alcohol is in itself a decisive role play in the arena of the communicable syndrome. The drunken identity seems closely related to the ghostly existence of the virus that shadows you if contracted.

The old man then comes back into the discussion by making an historical comparison: 'In the old times old men drank, not young men. Nowadays young men can drink the strongest alcohol available.' A participant explains that some 'alcohol is very strong'. 'There are softer drinks like *uraka* and local *pombe*, but we also take *gongo*, which Kikwete [the current president of Tanzania, author's remark] has forbidden. Women also drink nowadays, ten at the same time in groups. So when everyone is drunk, the epidemic spreads. Now I am OK, but if I get drunk I would come after you and want to touch your breast and everything else. In the old days it was a pleasure, but nowadays it has turned into bad behaviour.' This comment, which assumed a first-person perspective and was directed to my female research assistant Delphine Njewele, is, of course, difficult to unpack, but it is fair to assume that men look upon the personal and social phenomenon of alcohol as an alleged reason to behave in risky and injurious ways. And if alcohol allows you to change your behaviour, then it seems to be a consequence, in accordance with the mentioned comment, that other people who drink, including women as a collective category, implicitly make allowances for a changed behaviour toward them. Unemployment and other factors of insecure livelihoods thus seem to be a cause of alcohol abuse, while alcohol is linked to a promiscuous lifestyle where health and social regulations are compromised. The interpersonal and societal limbo that ensues is of course quite hazardous for women since the whole scenario is dictated by men.

Interesting comments on the background of, and specific problems with, unemployment were being made in the group. Furthermore, a remark was uttered about the uselessness of warning young people against HIV and AIDS since they do not heed guidance from elders anymore. It is the current and future state of the community that interested me, however, so after a brief talk about past social and sexual regulations that confirmed an old matrilineal order without really saying anything about the security and health situation of that era, we asked the group to comment on the existence of prostitution in Mumbaka (despite that this topic was mentioned by a single participant). An almost ten-second-long silence followed, then the old man resumed his personal speech: 'I am an old man and only carry 200 or 1000 shillings. Young women says "*Vipi mambo, vipi mambo!*", when they hit on you. Should I get that young woman? You give her the money and sleep with her. And they have short skirts.'[24]

Everybody in the group seemed to agree with this characterization. A fellow man exemplifies in more detail: 'Ceremonies nowadays have a lot of women. Women are hunting for men. We just take them and sleep with them. They misbehave at initiation ceremonies and night dances.' This punitive stance is backed up in retrospective terms by the senior man: 'In the old days if you wanted something you got it from your father – clothes, for instance. These days youth are very greedy in terms of fashion. Women get men, have sex, and then purchase modern things.' Another one jumps in: 'Even mini-dresses. Men get crazy by that.' Finally, the 'young drunk' wraps up the talk with the following deduction: 'Women come with short skirts and say '*Vipi kaka!*', '*Vipi mambo!*', and you don't care about dying, you just give them your 500 shillings and have sex. If you go buy local alcohol and a group of females help you to drink, they want you. First you are shy, but after one glass...'

It is quite clear that the group gravitated toward a consensus by gradually supporting each other's discursive alignment of unemployment, alcohol, and sex as primary epidemic determinants. At the moment when they had consolidated their argument about economic vulnerability and the ensuing social limbo, they had already pre-empted the inquiry about prostitution by holding external factors responsible for risky behaviour. The volatile external factors not only include job markets and culture-historical changes, but also the women as a social category of transformation. Hence if the upshot of unemployment is abuse of alcohol, then the upshot of drinking is abuse of social relations. Throughout their line of reasoning, the male focus group in Mumbaka managed to keep their own responsibility at an arm's distance and at the end of that arm is a finger pointing to women as responsible agents of change in a world that now lacks a stable domestic life, kinship system, and social hierarchy.

So what did the women in Mumbaka have to say about this? Well, just by reading the suggestions for topics to discuss, one can immediately see that their perception of the local epidemic is more personal. Just like the men, the women did mention poverty, alcohol, dress sense, and unprotected sex as discrete epidemic risk factors, but the overwhelming determinant was prostitution, mentioned by four out of five women. So it was only natural to start the discussion with that subject. After brief laughter, an elder woman opens the conversation: 'Prostitution is caused by the behaviour influenced by pombe. If you put on tempting clothes, men will even rape women. That's how the epidemic is spread. Young girls who tempt men and seduce men don't care about the epidemic; it's an occupational hazard for them; it's like a house fly to be killed at the wound. It's just normal.'

It is interesting to see that alcohol once again takes over the opening comment – it seems to be the primary social determinant in Mumbaka. And yet alcohol *per se* does not necessarily disclose anything about the decisive responsibility of a sexually transmitted epidemic; it is not like the parasite carried and transmitted by mosquito, but a concocted drink that is predicted to lead to sexually careless actions. As mentioned above, men know very well what will happen when they drink and they drink anyway. This is partly due to a relinquished sense of responsibility, which men ascribe to external factors such as economy, culture, history, but also women. In one sense, the old woman of the female audience group reconfirmed this view by pointing to the risks of drinking alcohol, dressing provocatively, and behaving nonchalantly. In another sense, though, the attribution of responsibility is very much a shared affair. If women act carelessly 'men will even rape women'. This is not the same thing as saying that women run the risk of contracting HIV if they simply have casual sexual relations. Another participant continues this discussion: 'Women always go for the men who have bought plenty of alcohol; so you find a group of men and you start to get drunk. They have sex in big groups. It may be 20 men with one woman.' The responsibility is, again, pointed to women who act recklessly, but this is said in relief against a quite brutal backdrop. It harks back to the comment made by the young female three years earlier in Mubaka about the woman who tempts men to have sex with her in a pombe place. And it certainly indicates the accuracy of the rehearsal in the youth centre three years ago.

The discussion dies down for a while, so I take the opportunity to ask an interview question, namely about the reason behind prostitution. A woman reflects back in time: 'We had prostitution in the old days, but it's much worse now. A girl can be in primary school and become house girls for wealthy or urban men and they are changed forever.' Then comes an older woman's confession, which could very well motivate an interpretation in a chapter of its own: 'In our days we engaged in prostitution, but there was no AIDS epidemic then (*lakini hapakuwepo ukimwi*). In these days, God is angry and tired of people and has sent a bad disease that cannot be cured, because they are not faithful to their spouses. I enjoyed prostitution in my days, for there was no AIDS. We could do it freely, without fear.' It is not entirely clear what this utterance actually asserts, but it does expose a cultural order where sexuality has been used as a social refuge from an unfeasible domestic situation. At this point, something happens in the group. It is as though we are getting closer to a painful truth behind the public discourse on poverty, alcohol, promiscuity, and morals – touching upon a culture-historical volatility and personal insecurity which has had to be coped with by clandestine means, long before AIDS came along. The group quiet down again. In an attempt to keep the discussion alive, I take the opportunity to ask an interview question about unfaithfulness in the community. 'Instead of staying home and being faithful while my man is being unfaithful', replies a woman, 'I just go out and find a man too. So we all go out and get AIDS.' The atmosphere is now slightly ill at ease. Delphine asks if anyone would like to add anything before we break up. Yet another discussant takes the opportunity: 'Poverty is also a factor. A woman thinks: I don't have money and a man from Dar es Salaam has money. Why should I refuse and starve? No, even when we know that this man is HIV positive, we would go with him if he has money.' This comment concluded the discussion and quite pertinently wrapped up my three visits to Mumbaka, but also prompted a need for interpretation of the cultural events I had witnessed as well as the speech acts I had heard.

The rationale behind the decision to conduct FGDs after performances was to assess the efficacy of CBT as HIV prevention. The rehearsal in Mumbaka youth centre in July 2003 was a simple piece that mixed generic HIV preventive counsel with site-specific risk behaviours. I do not know how many of villages in Marika ward the eventual performance visited, but I do know that it was accurate insofar as it dramatized the most frequently propounded determinant in the FGDs as a leitmotif, namely the abuse of alcohol in informal drinking places. The young people chose to foreground a leading character with mannerisms that were later anecdotally ascribed as pivotal triggers in the local epidemic, namely a young drinking man with money. Under the influence he listens to no one and walks away with one woman after another to have sex without protection. It is astonishing to notice the similarities between the dramatized young man and the so-called 'young drunk' from the FGD with the male Mumbaka audience. Hence the ostensive characteristics and other mimetic features in the work-in-progress were indeed realistic. The problem with AIDS in Mumbaka is, however, that realistic correspondences between the performance and the social order do not necessarily capture the real crux of the epidemic, since the latter is mainly impelled by invisible, taciturn, and other implicit factors. The imperceptible virus is spread behind people's curtains or in aloof heterotopia, gives rise to ghostly diseases and is mainly transmitted by means of untreated, and thus undisclosed, sexually transmitted infections. But the most significant determinant of AIDS, which turns it into an epidemic, is a social affair sanctioned in lopsided gender relations. FGDs serve to make the relations between the culture-historical arena of human interaction and the unnoticeable medical factors of AIDS perceptible and sensible. In other words, it points to a mimetic drama beside public campaigns and medical programmes. This is, of course, also what CBT is meant to do in public. However, the more discrete FGDs also serve the derivable purpose of indicating that CBT may be right about what it is doing and yet ineffective as HIV prevention. This was not my intention when I initiated FGDs in my research project; the aim was simply to acquire a more comprehensive understanding of the personal, performative, and societal relations of local epidemics. I did not foresee that FGDs would be a methodological tool for the assessment of CBT. What became clear, however, was that FGDs and CBT could say the same things and yet the public appeal of the performances would not necessarily further the aim of rallying a community against AIDS. Hence there seems to be something about the performative outreach component that does not take effect. Let me try to explain this in more detail before I resume the discussion about gender impeded culture-historical regimes.

AIDS is a recent phenomenon that has actualized old predicaments. Suddenly, these dormant predicaments threaten the future health of vast populations. In a deductive manoeuvre, then, one may find it problematic to apply contemporaneous countermeasures, such as CBT, against an epidemic that is driven by entrenched behaviours and inherited lifestyles. A performance such as the one in Mumbaka may very well be viewed as an event about a recent medical crisis that should be prevented by superimposed modern means like condoms, a morally sanctioned faithfulness, and a religiously motivated abstinence. In peripheral villages like Mumbaka, where one finds unique mixes of local traditions, Christian dogma, and modern lifestyles, these measures may not even come near the critical issues of AIDS. The ABC model, which obviously informed the script behind the rehearsal in the youth centre, is a contemporary concept that is, and always has been, controlled by men and powerful institutions.[25] This brings me a step closer to an interpretation of the performative malfunction of applied theatre against AIDS.

It seems to be the case that initiatives to break the silence and bring clandestine risk scenarios into the light are not enough to make CBT efficacious as HIV prevention, even though it offers the only public appearance of such scenarios in many places. This contradiction indicates that something inept remains in the very basis, or the framework, of performances and their project format. I believe this contradiction can be detected in recent research on so-called Theatre for Development. On the one hand, the versatile formation and wide-ranging application has made TFD arguably the most celebrated genre in African theatre today; on the other hand, this support has been tainted by a mistrust of its efficacy due to a constant dependency on national and international funding by organizations and agencies with special interests. An analogous contradiction can be found in the post-colonial attitude to performance on the whole in Tanzania. The performing arts, spearheaded by the nation's great variety of ritual dance (*ngoma*), represented a pre-colonial legacy in Tanzania which President Nyerere himself called to be revived with the help of cultural workers. The nostalgic notions about a pre-colonial national theatre has been radically questioned in the light of the commandeered deployment of cultural performance troupes for political purposes as long as Tanzania was a one-party state, and, more recently, the sparse public funding for the performing arts in the educational system, as opposed to its celebratory symbolic use in official functions such as during Independence Day. The fissures of the mentioned contradictions can be traced all the way down to the village level of Mumbaka. The implications of the contradiction do not pertain to the performative element of theatre as much as the acknowledgement of theatre. Apart from the ambiguous legacy of theatre as cultural performance it is worth considering that it is young people who are deployed to open and lead communal discussions on the taboo-laden topics around AIDS through performance. I am convinced that the key development of applied theatre today has to do with acknowledgement.[26] Let me concretize the issue of acknowledgement by redirecting it toward the rehearsal in Mumbaka.

According to the focus group discussions I conducted after seeing the performance in question, it seems clear that the epidemic in Mumbaka is thriving on impoverished and socially unsafe women who sell their bodies to drunk men with money who refuse to use condoms. To gear the play in Mumbaka toward the issues of stigmatization and discrimination of HIV-positive people, as was the case in the final scene of the rehearsal, seems to be an officially correct preference to address a generic problem with AIDS in accordance with the list of items that organizations like UNICEF put together in their standard leaflets.[27] But this key scene can be interpreted another way since there is arguably more to it than meets the eye. What we hear is a defeatist stance on holding yet another political meeting that will lead to nothing but the usual setbacks. The frustration then spills over into a diatribe against an HIV-positive man, a hostility that is picked up by the group of people, who eventually agrees to split up and cancel the meeting on the spot. A conventional way of understanding this collective breakdown would be to claim that the poverty stricken situation makes people so frustrated that they start picking on the weakest individuals in society, such as HIV-positive people. Another interpretation of the communal collapse would be to see it as a more self-critical event by reversing the state of affairs and suggest that the unsolved problems behind the AIDS epidemic, which the frustrated man gets reminded of when seeing the sick man, is in fact a cause of the political defeatism in the village. If the gender-infected determinants of AIDS can be traced back through the cultural practices and historical narratives in places like Mumbaka, then poverty does not necessarily qualify as the root cause behind the epidemic, but as a secondary cause behind a social division of labour, economy, and sexuality.

It is not clear whether the mentioned ambiguity was a conscious or unconscious reflection of the group, let alone whether it eventually generated post-performance discussions along the mentioned interpretive lines, but regardless of this the open-ended drama points to a highly interesting vicious circle. Again, it has to do with a domesticated gender politics of economy whereby women are living in a permanent extreme poverty while men may live in moderate poverty, at least periodically, which means some extra money to spend. This is especially disturbing since Mumbaka, like Likokona, is traditionally matrilineal and a place, like most other places in East Africa, where women commonly work much more than men in the agricultural sector. The inference of this complex scenario would be that many men seem to be engaged in extra-marital sex with the surplus of money that their wives have brought into their household through hard labour in the fields.

## A wider epidemic pattern

The rehearsal in Mumbaka youth centre showed the tip of the iceberg of the mode of epidemic spread and its culture-historical rationale, but that indicative semiotics is probably enough to stir up a debate in performance events among community members who are well aware of, but reserved about the hidden dimension of the scenarios. The scene with the hard-hitting drunk man who has unprotected sex for money with multiple women is, of course, not only indicative of the social conditions of Mumbaka, but in many other places in Mtwara and Mangaka districts (and elsewhere in Tanzania). It would not be meaningful to speak of the Mumbaka case unless it served as an example of a wider epidemic pattern. The fact that the man who was put at centre stage in Mumbaka was the one who assumed the female role of having multiple sex partners over one night does not mean that the more peripherally depicted women did not also have multiple partners. (It would be interesting to pursue an interpretation of the man with multiple partners in terms of a nostalgic behaviour of an inherited but obsolete kinship custom of polygamy, but that lies outside the scope of the present analysis.)

What was previously mentioned as a 'double act of upfront challenge and private resistance' on behalf of young women in casual relations turned out to be not only a consistent pattern of epidemic determinants in the district, but also an analogue to the public and confidential nature of community performances and FGDs respectively. In daily life, women do not always have the power to say no to unprotected sex; in performance, they can express such power but without a given social or political mandate; and in FGDs, they talk about condom use but without a public appeal. This is a problem not of awareness of AIDS or of an willingness to break the silence about it, but a problem of powerlessness due to a null and void official mandate. Young women represent the weaker sex in their homes, in schools, in public spaces, in organizations, as well as in performance. In the light of the epidemic profile of Mumbaka that crystallized through the mentioned rehearsal and the subsequent FGDs, this weakness translates into a vulnerability within the social dimension of the AIDS epidemic and thus a susceptibility to the bodily transmission of the HIV virus.

When I asked the audience focus groups in 2006 if they had seen the local group play theatre about AIDS, not one single discussant had seen a performance. However, the fact that CBT can fall short due to weak public staging in terms of official backing and that it may be viewed as a new form of communal intervention does not mean that it should be discarded as HIV prevention. Even under such circumstances, theatre still provides a unique opportunity of education and life skills exercise for young people; it still makes unseen and unmentionable scenarios accessible in public; and it is, not least, a diachronic and syncretistic mode of cultural performance that draws on ritual practice, culture-specific stories, dances and songs, as well as new, contemporary themes by means of international forms of participatory theatre. As opposed to naive notions about CBT as an application of self-sufficient and rapid problem-solving mechanism in cross-cultural conditions, I would propose that it should become even more closely aligned to local ways of living and governing. This double move suggests a simultaneous bottom-up and top-down approach. I will save the discussion on such advancements to the final chapter. But without appropriate political or organizational backing CBT is not acknowledged as a legitimate mediation in Tanzanian communities and, as long as it is not acknowledged as such, it will become a mimetic reflection of an epidemic condition where women continue to be insecure second-class citizens and men go on as agents of a doomed culture-historical potency.

# 4
# A Deadly Paradox: Assessing the Success/Failure of Community-Based Theatre against AIDS

Assessing the efficacy of community-based theatre as HIV prevention entails what could be called a deadly paradox: in the previous three chapters, one case after another shows that the ultimate accomplishment of this art of survival may be tantamount to failure. It may also be the case, *mutatis mutandis*, that many HIV prevention projects in Africa have succeeded in fulfilling their own stated goals and yet had no effect whatsoever on the epidemic. These inferences hinge on two pivotal and potentially contentious notions: first, the communicative routes of the epidemic and, second, the capability of theatre to identify and disrupt such routes. At face value, theatre *ought to be* the most auspicious mode of HIV prevention since its instantiation is so similar to the social situations whereby the virus is acquired. This was the hypothesis of the research project in the light of a number of stipulations. And if it is possible to identify the ghostly virus and its intersubjective communication, then it also ought to be possible to show and tell how it is possible to counteract the HIV incidences. With a retrospective through the previous chapters, the assessment of theatre has been broadened to consider its culture-specific pertinence and democratic potential as HIV prevention; CBT has, moreover, been recognized as a mode of intervention in a crises, with methods adaptable according to social predicaments rather than an invariable ritual regulation; furthermore, it has been distinguished as a form of performance that brings out back-stage issues of the most susceptible epidemic cohorts to deal with them in dialogue with the general public in local circumstances. Despite the timeliness, suppleness, and prowess of CBT, however, it would be naive not to say mistaken, and thus a great disfavour to its performers, to say that CBT is logically effective as HIV prevention. For that to be the case, the performers as well as the outcome of their action research would have to be taken much more seriously by organizations, agencies, coordinators, and leaders. The assessment therefore shifts over to another register of research, namely one about the political limits and possibilities of implementing effective HIV prevention at all.

The pandemic, which used to be viewed as a medical issue but which is now, more sensibly, considered as a chronic societal and political condition, has exacerbated notorious concerns like poverty and health care on a continent that already lagged behind the rest of the world for decades in these areas.[1] The pandemic has undermined institutions that people rely on such as education, marriage, political functions, judicial bodies, kinship systems, ritual regimes, and faith-based organizations. It took many countries, Tanzania among them, about twenty years to acknowledge that the key determinants of AIDS hinged on social relations rather than biomedical conditions or informational stipulations. Along with the abnormally long time of the asymptomatic infection, the culture of silence on sexuality, disease, and death makes the epidemic exceptionally hard to control. Reducing the understanding of the epidemic to medical and informational matters has given national authorities and the international aid industry reasons to sustain their discrete developmental programmes and discourses. Monetary and educational aid projects are, of course, much easier to control and quantify than 'soft' cultural programmes with local ownership over projects geared by critical inquiries, action research, and suggestions of long-term changes in social behaviour and gender relations. The latter approaches have no translation manual for efficacy *vis-à-vis* results to be readily displayed in glossy pamphlets with succinct results on behalf of international aid organizations, but require formative and continuous assessments by mixed means of communication, observation, and interpretation. There are no simple or rapid measurements to be done for gender trouble or existential fatalism, nor changes thereof.

The specialty of CBT is, of course, to operate by keeping a sharp focus on local states of affairs. Again, this seemingly auspicious quality can be perceived as detrimental if experts and authorities run ahead of themselves by looking for macro-political solutions to local challenges. In order to identify epidemic determinants within site-specific epidemics, HIV preventive projects must work as closely as possible with the social agents of the epidemic, preferably by direct involvement. This is the first of many ways in which theatre coincides with the impetus of AIDS. The relatively young social actors that drive the epidemic belong to the same cohort that takes the greatest interest in applied theatre and thus become theatrical actors. Mobilizing the most susceptible groups – for example, young uneducated men that hang around public hubs for labour opportunities and young uneducated women who work in the field and take care of domestic matters without much social esteem or public influence – are certainly not given participants in theatre projects, but since theatre group members are of the same age and background and consequently know the most susceptible individuals, the mobilization and referential scope of the performances do at least encompass them. In a group interview with gender-divided segments of the audience after a performance the dialogue turned personal:

*Man:*   Nobody knows how the youth groups are formed. We just see them at performances. We are worried that they are not the right people.
*Later another man asks:*   Is he [i.e., me] a donor of a group?
*Delphine Njewele (my research assistant):*   No, he is an independent researcher.
*Man:*   OK, if he is a researcher then he should hear the truth. The youth groups are not formed by the right people. When the authorities hear about a group being established, they go to the villages and pick their own relatives for the groups. This group is not functioning, unless someone comes and pays for them.

(Mpindimbi, Masasi district, 26 August 2006)

This piece of information may or may not be true, and should certainly not be interpreted as a general fact, but the matter of involving the most concerned individuals is a standing issue that  must not be underestimated in organized theatre. If a theatre group consists of exclusively talkative role models, it is highly likely that it misses some crucial epidemic predicaments, such as the taboo-laden, taciturn, marginalizing, and oppressive aspect of AIDS.

In the light of the intricate challenges to mobilize relevant individuals, capture the epidemic make-up within the format of community performances, engender post-performance discussions, and instigate follow-up programmes, it is fair to say that AIDS has driven African CBT up against its limits. Contrary to passé developmental discourses and clichéd academic jargons, there is, in my experience and opinion, no assurance about the facility of applied theatre to empower communal groups or change social life when it comes to AIDS. Applied theatre may, as Helen Nicholson (2006) writes, implicate a gift with ambiguous implications in Mauss's sense of the concept. On the one hand, it offers cultural participation with ample freedom of expression, but on the other hand, it is subject to highly uncertain exchange meanings and values in its encounter with target audiences. Certain kinds of applied theatre, such as community theatre, gives access to artistic research on matters which are as useful as they are painful to explore; the reciprocating response, when the times comes to do something about what has been scrutinized, is frequently one of achievement and further Theatre against AIDS may be seen as a gift that most people need but almost nobody wants.

## CBT as epidemiological counteraction

In an overarching epidemiological context AIDS can be said to have turned CBT into one of its symptoms, which is apparent in dramatic situations whose breaking points transgress liminal boundaries of ethical tolerance, existential attitudes, and communal actions. And if AIDS is a set of symptoms with social determinants, the real disease is a political syndrome of insufficient democratic opportunities for powerless people. In this chapter I will pursue a question that comes close to the political crux of AIDS, namely the lack of follow-up programmes in theatre projects. It is, of course, normally not advisable to investigate something non-existent, but in this case it is necessary for the assessment of CBT in the extended political field.

Before I go into greater detail in consequentialist analyses and recommendations, it is worth reminding the reader about some basic premises and *modus operandi* of CBT projects. The wider discussion of efficacy will also be preceded, just as in the previous chapters, by an example whose community event can epitomize and offer substance to the subsequent analysis. The critical research question was always quite simple: what is it, here and now, that causes the virus to spread from person to person, and from group to group? When the determinants, or risk factors, have been identified and mapped out by a local group on their home turf, attempts are made to identify the epidemic routes in virtue of people's shared experiences of social crises, their traditional ways of redressing cognate critical conditions, as well as their ability to take action against new crises.[2] To access and counteract the determinants behind AIDS it is necessary to mobilize the most relevant local individuals and civil society groups. These 'amateur experts' are aware of their own situational limits and possibilities, but are also ready to acknowledge a crisis without given empirical solutions or premeditated messages – unlike much previous applied theatre, such as the typically agenda-driven or task-based Theatre for Development. In the nationwide HIV prevention scheme launched by UNAIDS in Tanzania a few years ago (Mazzuki 2002), theatre projects against AIDS was viewed as a central part of the scheme, involving so-called 'community mapping', in which particular risk sites are ascribed stories of events informing a rough draft for eventual performances. The 'scripts' in amateur driven CBT are mostly verbally composed sketches and always leave a lot of space for improvisation. The scope of improvisation allows, in effect, for local variations in plots as troupes travel their own districts, where wards and villages in close proximity can typify quite disparate risk scenarios.

In connection to the community mapping and its allocation of narrativized incidents, daily routines and events are tricky to ventilate if they coincide with sexual affairs, not least extra-marital relations. It may, for instance, be guesthouses, marketplaces, or schoolyards that are viewed as the sites for casual or transactional sex; there may be unsafe paths for women fetching water at remote wells, or along smaller roads with sporadic traffic or other unreliable heterotopia. The most crucial epidemic hub, though, is the private household. Most spectators know about, or will at least have heard of, sexual relations in all of the mentioned loci and most people surely know about their own homes as a risk site. This is part of the alienation effect of CBT performances: to confront audiences with issues they are well aware of, but do not verbalize or act out in the presence of each other.

The community mapping converges with site-specific performances where spectators are aware not only of the intimate problems but also the local performers. By breaking the silence on issues like sexuality, stigmatization, disease and death, by exposing unseen affairs and private conflicts, disclosing the secret acts of initiation rites, casting doubt over religious dogma, embodying the bedridden in the dark corners of houses, and letting the vigil of family members of dying parents or children come into public view, the representational distance between actors and spectators collapses into performative acts – particularly in Austin's (1962) functional sense – where shows cut so close to the bone of matters that they become the matter. By enacting life-size situations in the public domain with, and for, directly involved social actors and performing the ailing and dying in broad daylight, the theatre stands in for former rites of afflictions on a par with current epidemic incidences. The countless numerals in statistical incidence and mortality rates come alive in events where one's spouse or next-door neighbour may turn out to be a typical representation of what otherwise appears as an outlandish scourge. Furthermore, the audience becomes an integral part of the blocking, as it were, of HIV preventive scenarios. To emphasize the participatory dimension, a Joker commonly steps into the breach of the open-ended plot and asks people what they are going to do. 'Was it a fair depiction?', 'Do these things happen among us?', 'And, if so, what are we going to do about them?' In other words the spectator gets reminded of his or her double role as theatrical witness and social player in the communal events. They also know that they have to act upon such appeals if they want to sleep comfortably that night.

It is interesting to see how community groups can situate the epidemic in their own communal time and space. In a Kenyana village near the Ugandan border in the Kagera region a group is still composing and performing songs that contextualize the epidemic outbreak in the early 1980s in detail:

> Come gather mothers and fathers [...] We now know that AIDS is the problem [...] It was first seen in Kanyigo village and then poured over the border at Mutukula [...] People didn't know and left behind orphans who became street children [...] Tanzanians and Ugandans thought they had bewitched each other [...] in 1981 doctors announced that it is a virus which weakens your immune system [...] AIDS is caused by sex [...] Please stop drinking and taking drugs [...] We urge you to change behaviour to survive [...]
>
> (Kenyana village, 19/03/2004; the cited phrases are taken from two songs performed at the occasion)

This is an example of how a historical record gets lyrically inscribed in a live storytelling tradition, invoking the communal reverberations of an incarnated 'we' on behalf of those who passed on (cf. the last phrase). It may seem as rudimentary information for people who already knows the risks and consequences of the epidemic, but it is in fact directed at new generations for whom AIDS is a brand new threat. For older generations, spiritual and narrative songs about the epidemic may carry a communal sentiment which brings them to tears. Somewhat in contrast to such lyrical compositions, propagandist political choirs hammer out more pragmatic advice for the purpose of proactive, protective, and collective actions. Both types of choirs often appear in similar styles in terms of costumes and movements. The aesthetic and technical consolidation has its pros and cons as it brings people together under the guidance of life-saving messages or admonitions, while it can also hinder fine-tuned dissidents or sub-cultural depictions of the epidemic onslaught.

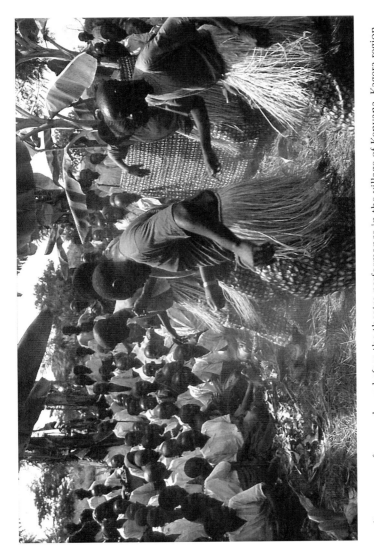

*13* A community group performs a dance before the theatre performance in the village of Kenyana, Kagera region (Photo: Ola Johansson)

The Joker in Kenyana poses his questions after the songs. The villagers remain quiet for a while. It is not just that a painful past has been unearthed and that pragmatic questions for action followed, a scorching sun also forces everyone to seek shade under the slender banana tree leaves. The local politicians and elders sit on one side, the schoolchildren are scattered on the ground, while the rest of the villagers sit around the temporary 'stage' area. In the background, quite significantly, is a primary school and a little further away the local government office. 'We should establish a fund for orphans', a man suggests in the local tongue Ruhaya. The Joker asks: 'How?' No one answers. 'Discuss it!' the Joker insists. After some muffled and stumbling exchanges, the Joker puts the matter on its head: 'Are we poor? Can we start a fund? How many work? How many can help with 500? 300? [Tanzanian shillings, about 20–40 US cents; my remark].' A man who presents himself as a mechanic says: 'God help me, I'm poor!' But a fellow spectator ripostes: 'We should sit down together and find a way. We are not so poor that we cannot help our children to go to school.' The Joker pushes that train of thought further: 'If you have 800 workers and they contribute with 500 shilling each, you would get 400,000. That's ten orphans in school!'

So far so good. The post-performance discussion lands in a promising plan for the local orphans. This kind of fund raising is something I have witnessed in other villages in Kagera region, where several hundred thousands of orphans are currently living and dying. It is also something which people should be aware of in the Northern hemisphere. No matter how much foreign aid a country receives, the overwhelming support for people affected by AIDS and other far-reaching crises is, and will always be, communal and, ultimately, familial (in Africa pertaining to so-called extended family systems).[3] Local donations for orphans are tremendously important, but not a test of what state-of-the-art CBT against AIDS can achieve since it exemplifies an instrumental response by a one-way communicative message and offers a temporary remedy to an enduring predicament. After the choir, the theatre ensues and things are about to get much more complicated.

## The multiple lives and deaths of Neema

A man comes back to his house after a long absence only to find his family in shambles. The mother has lost control over their two teenaged sons, who either keep fighting each other or smoking opium in their ragged clothes, probably out of the boredom of being stuck between disrupted schooling and permanent unemployment. The older brother barely takes notice of his homecoming father, not even when he is handed a gift from him. It is obvious that the father tries to re-establish his authority as head of family by material means. This is seen as futile by the older brother who soon picks a fight with him.

The paternal role has less than decent traits. As soon as the father is left alone in the house, he calls out for the housemaid Neema. In a softened voice, he addresses her as his daughter. In that personal vein she takes the opportunity to ask for a pay raise. He says she will indeed get something extra and drags her into a room – a booth covered with cloth in the middle of the play area – where he has sex with her. As so often during such scenes, the audience emits a scattered and embarrassed giggle. The sex scene is then repeated when the older brother forces Neema to have sex with him in the same place, and then threatens her to keep quiet about it. The audience giggles again. Like a farce, the scene is then repeated again when the younger brother coerces Neema to have sex. This time the audience laughs nervously as the farce turns into tragedy.[4]

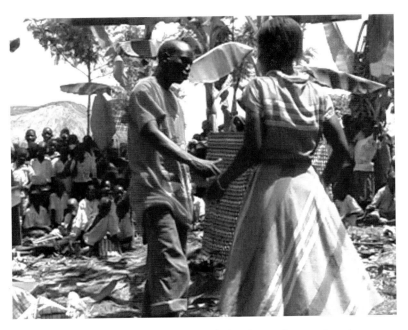

14  The older brother grabs Neema's hand after demanding sex from her
(Photo: Ola Johansson)

The rest of the intrigue is predictable although mordantly sad. A nurse visits the house – incidentally from Ndolage hospital where the first AIDS case in Tanzania was diagnosed in 1983 – and announces that Neema has just died from an AIDS-related disease. Panic whips the senses back to reality among the male family members. In a distressed state, the mother also figures out the plot and so the family that used to be only geographically disintegrated implodes into a jumble of social remains beyond remedy in their own home. Later a priest makes a visit and reads from Corinthians: '[...] now remains faith, hope, love, these three; but the greatest of these is love.' After the recitation, the clergyman grimly asks what happened to love in the house. It is a good question, but begs numerous other more or less related questions (which cannot be posed nor answered within the format of this article). One of the more provocative follow-up questions is whether a woman like Neema could actually afford real love in her lifetime.[5]

So what can an audience say after an in-your-face tragicomedy on AIDS? Well, everyone seemed to be taken aback by the straightforward depiction of sexual abuse. Before a word was uttered the children were escorted back to school. After a lingering silence – which is, of course, as telling as any discourse – a man suggests that the family in the play, just as families in real life, perished due to sexual greed. The spectator went on to say that this theme was merely mentioned in the songs, while the theatre made it a key theme. His remarks went uncommented, perhaps because it tapped into a religious discourse of cupidity and guilt that is too abstract to do something about on the spot. The next comment by a younger woman was also religiously correct: 'Being honest in your marriage is a crucial issue', she said, and added a warning against the use of drugs and alcohol. The truth is that the audience did not have too many things to say about the performance – the post-performance discussion soon stagnated and died out.

There are two major causes for the communicative breakdown in Kenyana, apart from the obvious fact that it is always awkward to discuss sexual matters in public (which is as true in the North as in Africa). First of all, in 2004 seeing a performance on the deadly impact by, and on, infected families as a result of AIDS was to arrive at an eschatological abyss between a defeatist rock and a deadly place. Taking an HIV test with a bad outcome back then could, at best, imply an altruistic act that gestured toward an individual behaviour change to save others' lives (cf. Reynolds Whyte 1997: ch. 9). This was, of course, several years after anti-retroviral medicines were introduced and made available for infected people in the Northern hemisphere. Today ARVs

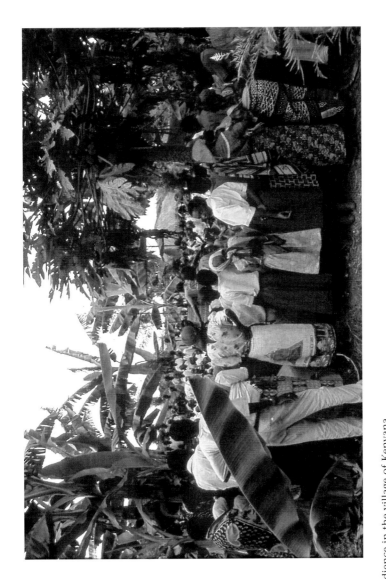

*15* Audience in the village of Kenyana
(Photo: Ola Johansson)

are available in selected hospitals in Kagera region, such as already mentioned Ndorage, which does not mean that more than a fraction of the sick actually gets access to therapy. According to epidemiologists Gideon Kwesigabo (interview 29 May 2007) and Stefan Hanson (2007), predicted scenarios show that only about 25 per cent to 30 per cent of the sick will get access to ARV therapies in the near future.

The other cause behind the communicative breakdown in Kenyana is more complex and has to do with a problematic mix of social and ethnic traditions, patriarchal supremacy, generational discrepancies, and other gender-related predicaments. Yes, I do generalize the complex of problems by pulling together a range of historical and culture-specific issues in terms of gender inequities. This is what science is about: finding related causes behind symptomatic issues. But in this case, it is not a matter of boiling down a deductive theory to explain reality, but an inductive procedure whereby a series of different, and sometimes contradictory, cases can be interpreted as cognate exemplifications of a particular phenomenon, namely how HIV is contracted through sex in situations where women, especially, do not act out of pleasure or other voluntary incentives. Women are not, however, the only subjugated gender cohort under the current epidemic conditions, but they do share some risk scenarios with the general stratum of young men. Young men and women – more than half of the population in sub-Saharan Africa are under 20 years of age – are the most susceptible strata in the African AIDS pandemic and, not coincidentally, the ones who make most use of CBT. The reason for this is that CBT arguably is the most democratic response to the most serious democratic challenge for decades in African countries (cf. de Waal 2006). Young people are open for identity formation and therefore clash with older and more obstinate spectators (Klink 2000).

A play performed the same week (11 March 2004), in the same district as the Kenyana performance, presented cognate predicaments. In Ijumbe village a group enacted the cruel exploitation of a housemaid trapped in the same tight spot as Neema, that is, the double bind of having one of the rare wage employments available for young rural women in Tanzania at the price of having a sexually abusive employer. Many poverty stricken women find themselves forced to become sex slaves, not least if they have children to support. In Ijumbe the vicious circle turned into a triple bind when an orphaned girl is hired as a maid by a businessman who takes sexual advantage of her. In a deeply moving story, it is the girl's alcoholic aunt who puts her up for sale and who ultimately becomes dependent on the girl as she falls ill from AIDS-related diseases. Abuse of alcohol is as commonly referred to as a cause of the epidemic as is gender abuse and is just as obviously linked to the underlying problem of poverty.

After the performance, the Ijumbe group put on a dance and a hymn for the vendors and visitors at a local marketplace. As always everyone enjoyed the upbeat *ngoma* and a few joined in. The dirge that followed about AIDS, however, caused nearly each and every man to turn back to their market activities. It is hard to say precisely what caused most men to steer away from the sombre choir, but it appeared to be a matter of priority, that the market activities became more important in the moment of lament. If so, it would serve as a metonymy of the gender roles which have become more and more evident throughout this study, namely that of the more outgoing and monetary male pursuits and the more domestic and caring responsibilities of women in contemporary Tanzania. It also reflects the preferences in the FGDs spoken of in Chapter 3, where women tended to put more emphasis on existing and familial concerns, while men were inclined to stress developmental issues. At any rate, it is probably the most evident gender divisive social gesture I have witnessed in connection with performances on AIDS and confirmed the importance of capturing young males in ongoing identity formations by means of theatre, before they are cast in this more mature masculine matrix.

Yet another similar plot was dramatized in Bugandika (10 August 2006), when a woman with a drinking husband takes her orphaned niece into her household. The village is located in a severely affected part of northern Kagera region – just a few miles from Kanyigo village that was mentioned as the epidemic fountainhead in the choir mentioned above – and, to the horror of the young woman, her auntie soon dies. At the funeral the drunkard husband begs the community residents for help, but despite his shaky state people deny him support since he always refused to cooperate with the village in their common funding for people in his present situation. Things go from bad to worse as the niece finds herself cornered in the man's house and ends up being raped. In the end, nearly everybody is found HIV positive (in light of the epidemic history of the village this is a quite realistic scenario). The suggested outcome is, again, fundraising for the orphan centre. This means that performances by three separate community groups share a thematic triangulation by typifying young poor or orphaned females as the leading roles in their action research on AIDS. Hence, understanding viable epidemic counteractions is not only a matter of widening the view from a medical perspective to that of a social horizon, but also of being able to focus in on quite distinct key roles and actors in social life.

Nelson Mandela has said that AIDS calls for a 'social revolution' (quote in Hansson 2007), a notion that may become feasible if, but only if, radically reformed gender roles are sanctioned to be the avant-garde in civil life.

In the case of the performances in Kenyana, Ijumbe, and Bugandika, the actors and spectators are up against a historical horizon with scenarios not only of colonial disruptions of societal structures, but also a domestic history of gender inequity where the pre-colonial Haya kingdoms used tribute systems of slave girls (later encouraged by German colonialists) and where women in post-colonial times have found themselves driven into systematic prostitution in order to cope with a lack of inheritance rights, land rights, and other civil and human rights. In her excellent book *Women in Development: A Creative Role Denied?* (New York: St. Martin's Press, 1984), Marja-Liisa Swantz writes a well researched chapter on the culture-historical situation for Haya women and draws the conclusion that:

> prostitution has been the Haya women's response to the conditions which have too often treated the woman as an inferior being, a commodity of exchange, a tenant and a servant who could be dismissed at the will of the husband, and used for producing children who were then stolen from her.
>
> (Swantz 1984: 76–7)

Despite recent legal reforms, the hierarchical, polygamous, and patrilineal legacy of traditional Haya societies is still quite obvious in Kagera.

The democratic relevance of CBT against AIDS has to do with substituting health issues for ideologically fettered political agendas and religious dogmas. Ethical and political issues are no doubt intricately linked with health, but in my opinion issues of life and death outweigh dichotomies like right or wrong, or the political left and right. Brecht knew that when he formulated the motto, 'food first, then morality' in *The Threepenny Opera*. CBT is – or should be – an open-ended mode of action research rather than a norm driven deployment of ideological, pedagogical, or other special interests. The inductive exploration of epidemiological conditions does not lend itself exclusively to written research or lab practice so much as it extends also to people with local knowledge and life skills. If action research is allowed to function on a culture-specific level, it can flesh out vital features and distinctions in risk analyses that otherwise get diluted when issues are elevated to a conceptual, institutional, or other type of generalized level of reasoning.

One of the most common generalizations in discourses on AIDS in sub-Saharan Africa is the view that poverty is the root cause of the spread of HIV. Needless to say, there is some truth in this argument but it is, nevertheless. vague; it does not serve very well as social analysis or cultural interpretation, and it is not practically adaptable in preventive interventions. Action research such as CBT does not bring closure to inquiries by quantifying issues, it keeps processes and outcomes open as long as social actors are working out issues. All too often in social research on AIDS there is the risk of an epidemiological fallacy in the sense that investigations merely map out and descriptively enumerate risk factors, whereby numerous small truths may add up to one big lie, namely the idea that AIDS is an infinitely complex and permanent quandary. But that may very well be a reflection of the scientific mapping exercise as such. AIDS is about the routines of daily living and livelihood; the question is how the routines can be opened up for discussion and plausible change between spouses, neighbours, teachers, politicians, religious leaders, elders, parents, and children. It is about social relations within and between public institutions and domestic regimes. CBT takes epidemiological and other quantitative research into account – many places in Africa are full of facts and rumours about overwhelming incidence rates and prevalence trends – but instead of leaving matters on a descriptive level or aiming for explanatory closure, applied theatre is enacting facts, accounts, and stories through performative means that show and tell audiences how actions can be transposed from action to interaction and, ultimately, to counteraction. Poverty can be counteracted if household economies as well as property and land rights are treated not as abstract, historical facts, but as man-made contemporary predicaments.

After witnessing more than a hundred CBT performances on AIDS in Tanzania and other places in Africa in recent years, I have identified the most consistently depicted determinant of HIV/AIDS as gender discriminatory household economies and their links to transactional sex. In fact, performances on gender issues do not even have to allude to AIDS for the audience to understand what danger it poses to young women in the epidemic. I saw a simple performance in Masasi town (17 July 2003) in which a woman gets so frustrated over her domesticated and impoverished situation that she physically attacks her husband. It soon turns out that he spends their money on a second wife (a so-called *nyumba ndogo*) in another house. There was no mentioning of AIDS in the show and yet every spectator knows which kinds of risk a situation like this implies in terms of health.

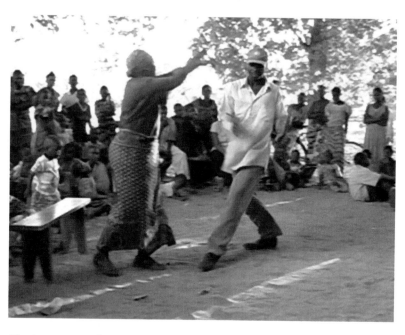

16   A woman pushes a man after finding out about his second wife; performance in Masasi town, Mtwara region
(Photo: Ola Johansson)

Almost all of the groups and performances that the research project
has examined have revealed clear examples of unequally distributed
poverty. In the focus group discussions and interviews with group
members and spectators of the performances, it has been uncommon
not to mention poverty as the cause of the epidemic. It is just that
when men speak of poverty, it is job related or even macro-politically
argued against, whilst women generally speak of poverty as a familial
predicament. Hence, the discourse of poverty is in itself indicative of an
entrenched deadlock to the solution of poverty insofar as it is ingrained
behind the institutionalized gender divisions of the private versus public, submissive versus assertive, protective versus proactive.

## Towards a community-based theatre as a relational agency

AIDS has brought with it the greatest democratic challenge in Africa
since the time of independence. It is a bodily syndrome that breaks
down a person's immune system, but it is also a societal set of symptoms

that weakens any community's immunity to critique. This may seem like a far-fetched analogy between a particular corporeality and a general order of things. In terms of a communicable disease, however, HIV is a virus that always runs the risk of spreading if the right to one's own body and mind is violated in a certain society. This applies not only to the current African state of affairs, but also to local governments, religious authorities, educational systems, non-governmental organizations, and (post-)colonial ramifications of global trade policies. There is no way around this complex body of influences so long as one identifies the cultural contexts of the disease.

As a complex cultural syndrome AIDS has forced CBT to go beyond, on the one hand, the notion of rapid conflict solving with target groups on specific developmental tasks and, on the other hand, the idea of a more basic awareness for those directly involved with theatre. The syndrome challenged the culture-historical limitations of CBT by urging it, according to theatre for development researcher David Kerr, to focus on 'sexual issues previously thought of as taboo', 'attitudes to women and children', and 'issues of human rights and social exclusion'.[6] In effect, once theatre practitioners recognized and counteracted the intricate epidemic challenges, they also challenged the limitations of current HIV-prevention projects by bringing them out of the medical realm of white-collar edification to the public arena of participatory practices, where alternative life skills are enacted by community residents. I do not believe it is a coincidence that the two Tanzanian regions (Kagera and Mbeya; see Kwesigabo 2001 and Jordan-Harder 2004 respectively) where decreases in AIDS prevalence trends and HIV incidence rates have been recorded have had an abundance of active theatre groups involved in AIDS control programmes.

It is not possible to change an epidemic by either discrete performances or projects or with an ideological awareness as such. The epidemic challenges have brought about typological as well as functional consequences for the theatre. The typological consequence has to do with the historical trajectory of community theatre, from its didactic foundation in colonial times to its autonomous formation in post-colonial times, which again needs to be unpacked, re-evaluated, and rewritten as a cultural practice. Sustainable self-reliance is a vital condition for groups who are fighting for free speech and the liberty of association, but the naive notion of artists as 'floating islands' (cf. Barba 1986) can also be an isolating factor if the task is about wider issues than the endurance of theatre groups. The functional consequence has to do with strategic objectives other than change. With associations to political 'revolution' and 'self-determination', the practice of CBT has come to define itself as an 'alternative practice', and 'the end point to this exploration of the alternative, and the "other" as an instrument of alienation and subjugation, is to seek a point of equilibrium or change' (Kidd 1973a, b; Salhi 1998; Abah 2002).

The course of actions as planned and implemented in theatre against AIDS should not aim for change *a priori*, but rather function as a critical examination – a form of comprehensive action research – of the conditions for people to lead healthy and constructive lives. Communal intervention becomes necessary in generalized epidemics, so it is not a matter of group dynamics as in drama-in-education, drama therapy, or so-called process drama (Simpson and Heap 2002). Theatre activities should bond and bridge social capital within and between groups (Campbell 2003: 55–8; Putnam 2000). The debate about political self-determination versus donor affiliations is an old one for community theatre, as well as for civil society groups versus governmental influences (Kerr 2002, 1995; Kasfir 1998). Discursive and economic self-reliance is, of course, important as resistance to post-colonial didacticism, academic elitism and authoritarian top-down projects, but once civil society groups working against AIDS have been established, they need to align themselves and coordinate their schemes with associated programmes. The argument I want to make and urge for more research around has to do with a fundamental revision of the idea of an efficacious community theatre, especially as pertaining to the AIDS epidemic and cognate complex crises, by emphasizing its crucial qualities as a relational means for change, a generic nexus in local peer-education programmes and comprehensive schemes in the public sector, rather than a means in itself or a means for rapid change. Theatre is, of course, a small device in the pandemic apparatus, a petty franchise in the big business of AIDS aid in Africa, but it is the link that can join the weakest parts in the chain of HIV preventive measures if aligned with relatable efforts. The performances I have referred to take place in public hubs of social life. A stone's throw from these performance grounds there will be one or two schools, a couple of churches, a mosque, a hospital, miscellaneous workplaces, community centres, a court building, a prison and various NGOs. In most places, none of these institutions or organizations invites young people's theatre groups, nor do they get encouraged by authorities to do so. When I revisited the 20 theatre groups that I first met a few years ago, it soon became clear that well-connected groups were still doing well (regardless of whether they were sponsored or not), while the more isolated groups were waning.

The AIDS epidemic is as serious as it ever was and will remain so for many years. New generations need to be offered opportunities for participatory life skills and peer-education programmes, they need to be recruited and to recruit peers to counselling and voluntary testing centres and thereby get access to the newly introduced anti-retroviral drug therapies, and they need to be taken seriously by politicians and other stakeholders. The time for pilot projects is over and it is high time for the realization of follow-up programmes in cooperation with schools, hospitals, people living with HIV or AIDS, elders, NGOs, governmental agencies, and so forth. A few serious programmes have been rolled out, such as the coordinated multi-sectoral approaches in a nationwide Tanzanian District Response Initiative (DRI) organized by the Tanzania Commission for HIV/AIDS (TACAIDS), in which Community Mapping and Theatre against AIDS (COMATAA) held a central place. But it is one thing to plan programmes in Dar es Salaam, and quite another to implement them at community level. Progress is constantly made on paper, but seldom *in situ*. At a meeting with TACAIDS (4 September 2006),

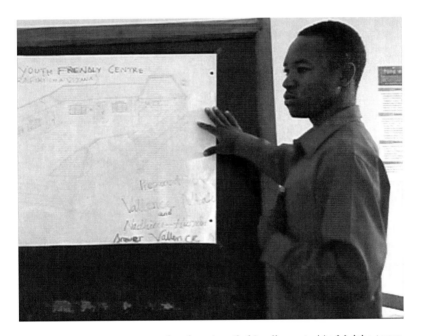

*17* A young man presents a plan for a 'youth friendly centre' in Muleba town, Kagera region
(Photo: Ola Johansson)

I was told that youth are represented in district committees in line with the DRI guidelines, but that their influence had not yet been evaluated. Still later (21 May 2007), I interviewed programmers from the same organization and they said that theatre will not be part of the new mid-term scheme (2008–12) for district responses to AIDS.[7] To this I want to say that they did not even try it out or evaluate it properly, but rather gave up the attempt.

The lack of evident progress in HIV prevention in Masasi district is having concrete effects on theatre groups. While many groups are doing well in the Kagera region, where the health-care system, youth centres, and governmental agencies are conducting coordinated work (at least in some places), things are worse in Mtwara region. Some groups have simply given up; on my random revisits three years after my initial fieldwork, most village residents I met confirmed that they had not taken part in theatre events for a long time, which usually indicates a general absence of prevention activities. In the village of Lukuledi (24 August 2006), a group presented a 'variety show' of old-style struggle songs, poetry, and speeches, obviously intended for visiting political delegations and potential donors. In the village of Mikangaula (29 August 2006), a remaining fraction assembled just to hear in a quite passive fashion what the *muzungu* (white person) had to offer them. I had to remind them that I am a researcher, not a donor. The already mentioned group in Likokona sang a highly ironic *shairi* (poem) in 2003 about failing UNICEF promises; three years later (28 August 2006) when I revisited, they were still highly interesting as they put on an innovative performance on the local epidemic scenario with a provocative ending for post-performance discussions. They had apparently stopped waiting for support at a certain point and managed to finance and organize their own activities. In Mpindimbi (25 August 2006), a youth group performed a meta-theatrical piece about seminars that people attend but forget about as soon as they get drunk. The thematic range of these performances suggests that the CBT in Mtwara is either vanishing or turning towards its own performative conditions of conducting HIV prevention.

## Recommendations

The findings of my research project indicate a war lost after victory in every battle. The studied projects in Tanzania mobilize the most susceptible epidemic cohorts and offer them participatory and gender balanced means to catalyse experiences, discourses, and life skills through local modes of traditional performance as well as contemporary international drama methods. The performances consistently attract considerable crowds who are exposed to, and often prone to share, taboo-laden topics and, at best, follow-up ventures. In FGDs with members of theatre groups as well as audiences, backstage perspectives toward risk scenarios consistently verify the validity of action research through performances by theatre groups. Rural young women repeatedly testify that theatre is their only access to public opinion and participation in the development of a sustainable and secure civil society. In interviews with villagers as well as programme directors, almost all who have come in contact with theatre perceive it as a serious and significant form of HIV prevention. Government representatives and non-governmental organizations usually praise its emotional and communicative impact. As opposed to economically or biomedically driven campaigns, however, the perceptible appeal and sensitive pursuit of theatre projects makes it akin to archaic ideas of female qualities. Few organizations or agencies have anything qualitative to say about the efficacy or real impact of theatre in the greater scheme of AIDS. Epidemiologists and politicians still quantify projects and programmes in terms of the reached number of people *vis-à-vis* estimated incidence and prevalence rates for areas of implementation, but seldom make qualitative evaluations of the need for interventions with culture-specific means for susceptible or subjugated groups. The most serious conclusion to be drawn from this is that even if an intervention driven by theatre were successful as an epidemic diagnosis and counteraction, it would not be noticed by project stakeholders, let alone policy-makers who collate and evaluate reports on AIDS campaigns.

The flip side to this dilemma is simply to presuppose the facility of applied theatre to change the order of things in which it intervenes, without recognizing the complexity of AIDS. The determination of change of course has its heritage in the revolutionary discourses and practical models of Freire (1971) and Boal (1979). Needless to say, any applied theatre project aspires to change. The question is whether change should be a built-in component or even a strategy of projects. Abah (2002) and many others predicate theatre for development on change by designing and assessing projects in terms of an alternative or new order. Thompson (2004), on the other hand, disengages this kind of requirement in what he calls theatre action research (TAR) by instead stressing how applied theatre can examine viable conditions for eventual community projects. Nicholson (2005) also leaves outcomes wide open, but by correlating applied drama projects with an abstract concept, namely the gift and its ambiguous claim and, every so often, paradoxical result in debt. With a slight amount of generosity, I could of course claim that the post-performance discussions leading to donations to orphans and widows in Kagera is proof of both an attitudinal and material change. Discrete and temporary changes, however, have little to do with the driving forces of AIDS. Real changes take effect through altered ingrained actions among people, not by what is given to them whether it is money, promises, or knowledge.

Another dominant but equally narrow view on efficacious theatre against AIDS finds justification in the concepts of information and education. Whilst an informative theatre mostly pertains to the transmission of medical or moral messages, educational theatre draws on the notion of drama as a pedagogical mode of telling and showing taboo issues. A crucial challenge thus lies in how to deal with the fact that people are as susceptible to HIV as ever, despite sufficient knowledge. It was therefore slightly disconcerting to pick up a supplement of the prestigious medical journal *The Lancet* on health and art, and to read a couple of articles on theatre against AIDS. Mbizvo writes that theatre is 'an effective and entertaining strategy for dissemination of health information and reinforcement of positive health messages' (Mbizvo 2006: 30; see also Klink 2000: 166). By effective she means that theatre breaks down communicative barriers for the sake of behavioural change, conveying knowledge about expected aid, and arousing audiences' 'emotions to stimulate acceptance of the messages' (Mbizvo 2006: 31). Rather than functioning as a mouthpiece for medical and political authorities, it is more relevant for theatre to show these people how and why their conventional strategies for communication, behavioural change, and biomedical aid have proven unsuccessful for the majority of people in Tanzania and most other sub-Saharan countries. And the only way to do this is to do what theatre does best: function as a revelatory and relational agency of young people's interests in cooperation with official agencies and non-governmental organizations that can meet and support such interests for the purposes of a worthy and safe life.

That young people enjoy the privilege of being backed by NGOs, however, does not always sit well with people who used to control public opinion. Ironically, the fair, unique, and independent features of CBT can also be a curse for its participants since such contemporaneous features have been licensed to young people from non-governmental organizations rather than earned through official merits (or favours). The groups can easily draw a crowd, bring spectators to laughter and tears, and provoke discussions, but without a mandate that provides the performances with a platform wider than the events *per se*, CBT will remain culturally alienated and not be able to effect social change.

Hence timeliness and unicity in design do not guarantee efficacy in performance. There are reasons to doubt a theatre against AIDS in the name of transformation, education, or donation. What, then, is it good for? If CBT engages the most susceptible epidemic target groups in participatory counteractions against risk scenarios in cooperation with communities, why is it so hard to speak of its efficacy? The only way to approach efficacy in CBT is, I believe, to identify its limitations and thus turn its insufficiencies under specific epidemic circumstances into reflective and productive forces. (Instead of celebrating applied theatre against AIDS, I believe it should be an obligation of researchers to highlight its problems, at least until it is possible to substantiate palpable achievements.) In the light of the findings of my research project, it seems obvious that the critical means and ends of CBT, which are so appealing and convenient to celebrate, neither have a recognized place in organizations that use theatre, nor a destination in societies where it performs. CBT does not have ownership over its own activities, often due to meagre financial means but even more so because of a deficient social legitimacy.[8] It is directly involved in precise epidemic problem solving and yet cut off, as it were, from epidemic-wide solutions. In Marxist terms, one may say that the groups are alienated from the purpose of their social work by being used as exchange items in the production of aid, rather than as useful agency in consequential prevention schemes. One of the most disturbing aspects of this problem is that the theatre facilitators from places like Bagamoyo College of Arts and (my Tanzanian host department) the Fine and Performing Arts Department at the University of Dar es Salaam which organizations use for their epidemiological and commercial purposes, never (not one I have spoken with!) receives feedback on their contribution to HIV preventive projects. The effect of the alienating division of labour is, again, that a potential achievement of theatre as HIV prevention would not even be recognized. If it is difficult to appreciate the effects of applied theatre, then it should at least be possible to see its obvious use as a means for young people to acquire life skills for a safer social existence. However, if the quest for efficacy is an epidemiological challenge, then the quest for a pragmatic use of it becomes a political challenge.

As Byam (1999) insists, the use of Boal's methods in theatre projects stands in need of an awareness of political frameworks such as those discussed by Freire to take effect in societal and developmental circumstances. The roles of the Brazilian pedagogues have been thrashed out in debates on African applied theatre since the 1970s, although mainly without much criticality. The reason why the discourse on theatre for development often stagnates is that it tends to hinge on certain celebratory concepts, such as radical change through theatre, the economical and political self-reliance of civil groups, and rapid appraisals of project efficacy. The discrepancy between the concepts and real political conditions is an interpretive gap that is often accrued by extending the methodological scope of Augusto Boal into the pragmatic visions of Paolo Freire. When individual or site-specific modes of understanding reaches the level of socially applicable self-reflection, as Freire points out, people enter into the realm of praxis where quite advanced attempts can be made to revolutionize policy making. In particular Freire's caution, with the backing of post-colonial philosophers like Fanon (1968), against unconscious identification with one's so-called oppressors, and the need to always uphold a critical dialogue about the means and conditions of liberating strategies, are invaluable pieces of advice for any CBT group.[9] However, in this publication I have mentioned project participants whose 'potential consciousness' has '[emerged] from reality' and who have already perceived 'the causes of their needs' (Freire 1970: 117). Through codified acts of problem-posing practices that are discussed in public (ibid: 122), they have indeed rehearsed their cultural revolution (Boal 1979: 141) through critical reflections and actions, attained ownership of their labour (Freire 1970: 183) and thus reached an entry point for an applied social performance of durable change. However, the fundamental need for CBT against AIDS has little to do with didacticism, utopian objectives, or radical policy; it has rather to do with an acknowledgement of already achieved cultural practices and their participants. The latter have attained 'conscientização' and are constantly, although casually, celebrated for it in quasi-educational terms. Given the lack of proper assessment, one may say that the theatre groups have created performances of effective communication, although without epidemiological efficacy.

Despite its clear pedagogical, organizational, logistical, critical, and intellectual merits, CBT is not allowed on to the arena of organized aid, public sectors, or real politics. Rather than just pointing to poverty and gender in sweeping arguments, the crux of the efficacy of theatre is its lack of legitimacy. This has not only to do with patriarchal communities resisting young people's creation of a new public opinion, but also with an unprecedented political challenge. It is a matter of democratic urgency to acknowledge that young people make up more than half of the population in Tanzania. This majority has more site-specific knowledge about the spread HIV than any imagined or authorized expert; they constitute the most susceptible groups in the pandemic; and they are the ones who make the most of HIV prevention practices through participatory means such as CBT. What they need is not a revolutionary breakthrough of utopian ideology or liberating knowledge, what they need is a performative democracy whose functions go beyond flags and polling stations, all the way down to the ground level of villages where most people in Tanzania pursue a reliable, healthy, and productive everyday life through acts rather than rhetorical declarations or judicial trials. That is the level and sphere in which a cultural legitimacy can be validated through actions. If CBT fails, or is allowed to fail by a deliberate neglect of its impact or recommendations, it is reasonable to assume that every other socially constructed form of HIV prevention also will fail.

CBT has the qualifications for functioning as a 'best practice' in HIV prevention and should be used as a relational agency in coordinated programmes.[10] It effectively attracts the core risk groups on a voluntary basis in the most AIDS-affected societies in sub-Saharan Africa; allows them to steep their popular views through ceremonial, ritual, theatrical, pedagogical, and informal/improvised modes of performance as well as through biographically and collectively informed community analyses; and in that way CBT meets the most urgent and taboo-laden issues head-on in performances and post-performance discussions where people, again and again, end up appealing to organizations and governmental authorities to consolidate actions in view of the depicted scenes. What the national district response initiative (DRI) in Tanzania needed when it rolled out was not only a poetic licence for young people to map out and depict critical behaviour patterns but also a political licence to apply its results in local programmes. It is difficult to understand why NGOs are willing to give community groups all sorts of education, except one in applied politics. In the interest of a more comprehensive democracy young people ought to be provided something like youth councils in local political offices. Meanwhile, it is unfathomable, not to say hypocritical, why authorities and NGOs in the districts where I have carried out fieldwork are not deploying voluntary community groups with responsibilities to, for instance: coordinate services like condom distribution out of hospitals; mobilize people for HIV tests and counselling under the aegis of ARV programmes; work in closer cooperation with schools,[11] faith-based organizations and workplaces; and, not least, be allowed to take on a greater role in the research, action, reporting, and evaluation of projects in cooperation with NGOs and AIDS coordinators. It is exciting to imagine what would happen if such a performative coordination and management, where words means action and vice versa, was in effect a political office aligned with community performances. The group in Kenyana who highlighted the situation for housemaids, the Likokona group that shed light on the link between corruption and AIDS, and the group in Bugandika who demonstrated the vicious circle for orphans, would have led not only to discussions and donations but also to enquiries and eventual reforms in communal, judicial, political, and educational systems. But this is, of course, exactly what authorities and NGOs do not want to happen since it would infringe on their agendas and audit books and threaten to take away their work. After having rehearsed their social revolution, to paraphrase Boal and Mandela in one breath, the community groups I have studied are now waiting at the point of entry to an official stage of politics where their democratic legitimacy is fully recognized.

# Appendix I

## Focus Group Discussions: *Modus Operandi*

Each youth centre selects 4–6 boys and 4–6 girls (in total 8–12 boys and girls) for focus group discussions. The daily programmes will be as follows:

(1) We introduce ourselves, hand over the video tape of the prior visit, and present the daily programme. It is important to indicate that the programme will take 5–6 hours to complete (including a break for lunch with the discussants). *(15 minutes)*

(2) We then ask the participants to formulate – or enunciate for those who cannot write – the *three most important issues to discuss* regarding the risks of being infected by HIV for young people in the present location. This should be done individually and confidentially, so that each participant feels free to express whatever he or she thinks is the most necessary issue to ventilate. The method of letting focus group members formulate the topics of discussions pertains to a method called 'question and answer' and aims for an optimum degree of participatory research. *(15 minutes)*

(3) After that, we collect the suggestions for discussion and keep the women's and men's suggestions apart. There should be roughly 15 suggestions for each group. Since some suggestions will coincide and overlap, we will need to sort out which of the suggestions will work best for the eventual discussions. It is important that this screening process is representative of the issues brought up by the participants. After this selection, there should be at least five topics of discussion points for the boys and girls respectively. The topics will most likely differ between the groups and should be kept separate. *(30 minutes)*

(4) Then we sit down – preferably in a place with minimum disturbance – with the first group (girls or boys) and allow it to discuss the suggested topics for as long as it takes to cover them. *(in all probability approximately one hour)*

(5) Then we do the same thing with the other group (girls or boys). *(about one hour)*.

(6) When the group discussions are completed, we treat the groups for a lunch break and eat together. *(one hour)*.

(7) After lunch we sit down with the groups together and discuss the different topics brought up in each group and how the topics and discussions differed between the women and men. *(1–2 hours)*

We end the sessions by assuring the youth centres that we will be back later with a summary of the discussions and with follow-up interviews.

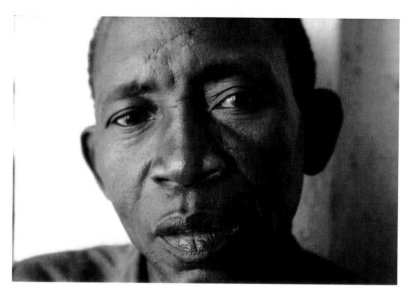

*18*   Mr Andrew Hamisi, a great friend and mentor, was the research assistant I worked with most of all during my research project in Mtwara region, as well as Dar es Salaam. Sadly, Andrew passed away in 2005
(Photo: Ola Johansson)

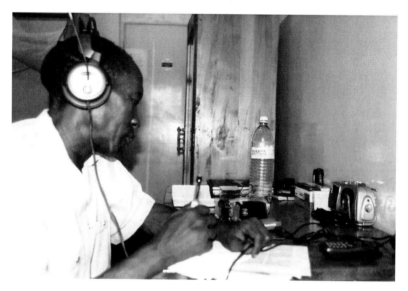

*19*   Andrew engaged in translation work in Dar es Salaam in 2004
(Photo: Ola Johansson)

# Appendix II

THIS QUESTIONNAIRE IS <u>CONFIDENTIAL</u> AND WILL ONLY BE USED FOR <u>ACADEMIC PURPOSES</u> AND WILL THUS NOT BE EXPLOITED COMMERCIALLY OR POLITICALLY OR FOR ANY OTHER REASON. I AM AN INDEPENDENT RESEARCHER, I.E., UNRELATED TO COMMERCIAL CORPORATIONS, NGOs, POLITICAL PARTIES, AND OTHER INTEREST ORGANISATIONS.

*Dr. Ola Johansson*
*Research Associate, Lecturer*
*Department of Musicology and Performance Studies at Stockholm University (Sweden)*
*Section of Theatre Studies, Lancaster Institute for the Contemporary Arts, Lancaster University (UK)*

Place & date:
...................................................................................................................

Name of interviewee (<u>optional</u>): .......................................................

Name & start year of organization:.........................................................

Sponsoring organization(s): ....................................................................

Cooperating organizations/preferred: ...................................................

Target group(s): .......................................................................................

How many people do you think carries the HIV virus?...............................
...................................................................................................................

1.  What is/are the goal/s of your organization?
2.  How would you like to see your organization develop? What are the major obstacles?
3.  Which are the major risk factors of HIV/AIDS in your district?
4.  Do you think you have prevented HIV transmissions? How do you report the results?
5.  Which methods of HIV prevention do your organization deploy?
6.  Why did you choose to use community theatre as HIV prevention?
7.  How have you used performing arts – e.g., plays, dance, choir, storytelling, poetry?
8.  What responses have there been to the performances (audiences, NGOs, political)?

9. **What kind of follow-up action has resulted from your projects? (fund-raising? IGAs?)**
10. **Specifically, what impact do you think community theatre can have on AIDS?**
PS. **Have I forgotten to ask you an important question, or would you like to ask me one?**

## Most commonly proposed FGD topics in *kagera*

| CATEGORY | % prop. | #prop. |
|---|---|---|
| Education | 17% | 49 |
| Poverty | 15% | 43 |
| Development | 8% | 24 |
| Alcohol | 7% | 20 |
| Unemployment | 5% | 15 |
| Children | 4% | 13 |
| Mortality | 4% | 13 |
| AIDS is getting worse | 3% | 8 |
| AIDS big problem | 2% | 7 |
| Counselling | 2% | 7 |
| Luxury | 2% | 6 |
| Sexual routines | 2% | 6 |
| (Un)faithfulness | 2% | 5 |
| Condom use | 2% | 5 |
| PLWHA | 2% | 5 |
| Medicine | 1% | 4 |
| Empower YC | 1% | 4 |
| Night dances | 1% | 4 |
| Prevention | 1% | 4 |
| Promiscuity | 1% | 4 |
| Prostitution | 1% | 4 |
| Sharp instruments | 1% | 4 |
| Uncertainty | 1% | 3 |

## Most commonly proposed FGD topics in *mtwara*

| CATEGORY | % prop | # prop. |
|---|---|---|
| Education | 14.5% | 47 |
| Poverty | 10.2% | 33 |
| Condom use | 9.9% | 32 |
| Alcohol & other drugs | 8.4% | 27 |
| Unemployment | 8.0% | 26 |
| Development | 4.9% | 16 |

(*continued*)

Continued

| CATEGORY | % prop | # prop. |
|---|---|---|
| Night dances/gatherings | 4.3% | 14 |
| Prostitution | 3.7% | 12 |
| Sharp instruments | 3.4% | 11 |
| Blood tests | 3.4% | 11 |
| Unfaithfulness | 3.1% | 10 |
| Circumcision | 2.8% | 9 |
| Polygamy | 2.5% | 8 |
| Abstinence | 2.2% | 7 |
| Trad. practices & beliefs | 2.2% | 7 |
| Inappropriate clothing | 1.9% | 6 |
| Desire for wealth ('luxury') | 1.6% | 5 |
| Multiple partners | 1.5% | 5 |
| Unsafe sex | 1.5% | 5 |
| 'Difficult life' | 1.2% | 4 |
| Public disclosure of HIV+ p. | 1.2% | 4 |
| Initiation ceremonies | 0.9% | 3 |

JQ 27/340/081/VOL 11?/DK26/155
SWEDISH
FG

"IMMIGRATION OFFICER"

17 AUG 2006

THE UNITED REPUBLIC OF TANZANIA

TIF 4B

The Immigration Act, 1995
(Section 20)

No. 00429:8

RESIDENCE PERMIT CLASS C

Mr./Mrs./Miss ...... SVEN OLA   MAGNUS JOHANSSON
P O BOX

is hereby authorised to enter Tanzania and to remain therein for a period of .... DALE TECH
.......... 15.19.1.200. for specific employment with COSTECH

and subject to the provisions of the Immigration Act, 1995 and to the following conditions:-
(a) (i)  Place of work ...... D SALAAM  BUKOBA MWARA
(ii)  Place of residence ......
*(b)  the holder shall not engage in any employment, trade, business or profession other
than ...... RESEARCHER

*(c)  wife and children whose names have been endorsed on this permit are not allowed
to engage in Employment ......
*(d)  (other specific conditions) NO CHANGE OF IMM STATUS

Description of Passport :-
Country of issue ...... SWEDISH            No. 52108217
Date of issue ...... 9.11.05          20 ......

Fees: US $ ...... 120 ...... received vide E.R No. 26694006 of 142.06
Issued at ...... DSM

All persons entitled to enter the United Republic under this permit must on entering the United
Republic report to an Immigration Officer without undue delay ( Reg. 18)

(Section 25)

17 AUG        Director of Immigration Services

| Full Name | Relationship to Holder | Age |
|---|---|---|
|  |  |  |
|  |  |  |
|  |  |  |
|  |  |  |

Date ...... 20 ......          Director of Immigration Services

*Delete if not applicable

# TANZANIA COMMISSION FOR SCIENCE AND TECHNOLOGY
# (COSTECH)

**Telephones:** (255 - 22) 2700745-6
**Director General:** (255 -22) 2700750
**Fax:** (255 - 22) 2775313
**E-Mail:** rclearance@costech.or.tz

Ali Hassan Mwinyi Road
P.O. Box 4302
Dar es Salaam
**Tanzania**

# RESEARCH PERMIT

No. 2006 – 242– ER- 2003–33                    Date: 24th July 2006

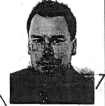

| | | | |
|---|---|---|---|
| 1. | Name | : | **Sven Ola Magnus Johansson** |
| 2 | Nationality | : | **Swedish** |
| 3 | Title | : | **Community Theatre as Preventive Intervention in the African AIDS Pandemic** |

4. Research shall be confined to the following region(s) **Kagera, Mbeya, Mtwara, Mwanza and Ruvuma**

4. Permit validity **24th July 2006 to 23rd July 2007.**

6. Local Contact/collaborator **Dr. Frowin Paul Nyoni, Faculty of Arts and Social Sciences, University of Dar es Salaam, P.O. Box 35044, Dar es Salaam**

7. Researcher is required to submit progress report on quarterly basis and submit all Publications made after research.

H. Gideon
**for: DIRECTOR GENERAL**

*21* Tanzanian Research Permit

# Notes

## Introduction

1.  In Swahili, the official language of Tanzania, AIDS spells 'ukimwi', an abbreviation of upungufu kinga mwilini, which is a rough translation of the English word AIDS, i.e., acquired (upungufu) immuno deficiency (kinga) syndrome (mwilini).
2.  The conference was called 'Language, Literature and the Discourse of HIV/AIDS in Africa' and took place at the University of Botswana in Gaborone, 24–28 June 2002, with sponsorships from UNAIDS and the University of Botswana. I presented the paper 'Performative Speech in African Community Theatre on HIV/AIDS'.
3.  For information about the video collection called Steps for the Future, see http://steps.co.za/ (accessed 11 April 2010).
4.  See http://www.aegis.org/news/sapa/2002/SA020409.html (accessed in August 2009).
5.  During that visit to Bukoba I visited a Swedish woman called Deborah Brycke, who has lived and worked in Kagera since 1969. Her organization, The Tumaini Children Centre, has a firm reputation of receiving orphans and accommodating them in centres and educational settings. When I visited, she introduced me to a young girl who had suddenly turned up outside her gate the day before. The girl said she came from Karagwe, a nearby Tanzanian district, but Deborah thought she may have come from across the Rwandan border a few miles further away. When it comes to migrating orphans, it is often hard to determine the cause behind the displacement. When it comes to AIDS orphans, it is, again, only possible to estimate their quantity and percentage.
6.  Cohen-Cruz, Jan, 'Practice & Policy in Theatre & Development', in Martin Banham, James Gibbs and Femi Osofisan, eds, *African Theatre in Development*, Oxford: James Currey, 1999, p. 115.
7.  Toolis, Kevin, 'Killer on the Road', *The Guardian*, 3 July 2002 (see http://www.guardian.co.uk/world/2002/jul/03/aids.kevintoolis (accessed 12 April 2010).
8.  *Sunday Observer*, Dar es Salaam, 23 September 2001.
9.  Later I was informed by my colleague Stephen Ndibalema, lecturer with the Fine and Performing Arts Department at the University of Dar es Salaam, whose wife is a secondary school teacher, that the vulnerability of teachers has to do with their low wages, which are in effect a result of very weak trade unions for teachers in Tanzania.
10. The Joker function of course comes from Augusto Boal's forum theatre. Many artistic facilitators in Africa, including Michael Kifungo, are aware of this role function and its source, even if they seldom manage to develop the Joker into the dynamic and role swapping agent that Boal instructed for a forum theatre event. Anything beyond an open post-performance discussion

amongst the audience and actors would be a tall order in local settings where AIDS is taboo-laden.

11. Michael Kifungo's group was instructed in forum theatre technique by Stephen Ndibalema from the Department of Fine and Performing Arts at the University of Dar es Salaam. Ndibalema, also from the Kagera region, later worked with me in the same region.

12. The documentary was aired on CNN and MTV on World AIDS Day on 1 December 2004 as part of a series of short films called 'Staying Alive'.

13. As will be discussed later, this is not as straightforward as it may seem, though. The Lutheran Church of Tanzania, like every other religious organization in the country, is against the use of condoms. The branch in Bukoba, however, seems to be wise enough to tacitly agree upon condom promotion as long as it is not done in their name. It appears to be a case of 'don't ask, don't tell', by means of a poetic licence. By including scenes of condom use in the documentary, the group 'came out' through a different media outlet, but the group has not suffered financial or any other detrimental consequences after the broadcast.

14. *Omutoro* is a so-called heroic dance designed to show allegiance to the chief among the Haya people in Kagera. In this society only men could be heroes with a mandate grounded in encounters like hunting and warfare (cf. Barongo 1998: 3–4)

15. Mtwara and the rest of southern Tanzania retain an immense reservoir of traditional (ritual) dances which are still used by local communities as well as urban dance troupes all over Tanzania (cf. Lange 1995: 54–5).

16. It is worth pointing out an anomaly in the depiction under discussion. The fact that the girl has become sick from an AIDS related disease so shortly after contraction, i.e., in connection with the pregnancy less than a year ago, is not realistic and must be looked upon as a fictional strategy for illustrative purposes. The incubation time between the HIV infection and the opportunistic diseases associated with a weakened immune system is about ten years.

17. The explanations suggested include not only out-migration but also 'poor nutrition and sexually transmitted diseases' (Seppälä and Koda 1998: 19). In the region, 'many women are childless while women with only one or two children are also common, despite the high level of divorces and remarriages. The infertility is partly induced by the prevalence of syphilis and chronic gonorrhoea. An additional source of low population increase nowadays is AIDS' (ibid.: 21).

18. Mlelwa, Hadrian Cosmas, *Food Shortage and Famine Problems in Masasi District: From Colonial and Post-Colonial Era (1895–1991)*. Doctoral diss. University of Dar es Salaam, 1992, ch. 4.

19. http://www.populationaction.org/Publications/Fact_Sheets/FS32/Population_Growth.pdf

20. To be accurate, one should always denote AIDS in Tanzania as a pluralistic variation of 'epidemics'. Hanson (2007b: 78) identifies 15 different epidemic levels in Tanzania, among which the differences appear in accordance with local or regional characteristics.

21. *FHI/UNAIDS Best Practices in HIV/AIDS Prevention Collection* (2001), ed. Bunmi Makinwa and Mary O'Grady: (http://www.fhi.org/NR/rdonlyres/

e3hmq5w4o542tmtlhi66rtwqijhfqqzgaspcwkc55f327e6dvdc5a2d5zwjd
bdhhl7mgw6bprtmhip/FHIUNAIDSBestPracticesreduxenhv.pdf (accessed
9 April 2010). This collection is revised continually, with reference to the
following six criteria in HIV/AIDS programmes: relevance, effectiveness,
efficiency, replicability, ethical soundness, and sustainability.

22. The chapter draws on my article 'The Lives and Deaths of Zakia: How AIDS
    Changed African Community Theatre and Vice Versa', *Theatre Research
    International*, Vol. 32, No. 1 (Cambridge University Press, 2007a).

23. The chapter elaborates the article 'Performative Interventions: African
    Community Theatre in the Age of AIDS', in Franko, Mark (ed.), *Ritual and
    Event: Interdisciplinary Perspectives*. London and New York: Routledge, 2006.

24. My fieldworks account as follows: the Mtwara region, Tanzania: 4 fieldworks
    (2002, 2003 x 2, 2006); the Kagera region, Tanzania: 4 fieldworks (2003,
    2004, 2005, 2006), and a documentary film on theatre against AIDS in
    Kagera 2004; Dar es Salaam, Tanzania: numerous research visits to the uni-
    versity, governmental braches, National AIDS Control Programme, archives,
    NGOs, etc.; Bagamoyo College of Arts, Tanzania: visits and interview ses-
    sions in 2001 and 2003; Addis Ababa and Bahir Dar, Ethiopia: 1 month
    project in collaboration with UNICEF; South Africa: visits to Eastern Cape
    (2002), KwaZulu Natal (2003), and Western Cape (2007); Kenya: several visits
    from 1996, to the Mathare slum in Nairobi and to the central highlands with
    reference to HIV prevention; Botswana: 1 visit to a conference, performances
    on AIDS, and hospital visit in 2002.

25. Chapter 3 is partly informed by my article 'Eschatological Field Notes:
    Community Theatre, AIDS, and the Fate of Informant D. in Ilemera,
    Tanzania', published in *Nordic Theatre Studies*, No. 19, 2007b; and partly
    by a paper called 'The Quest for an Efficacious Community-Based Theatre',
    which was presented at University of California, Berkeley, at the conference
    'African and Afro-Caribbean Performance', 26–28 September 2008.

26. The chapter is based on my article 'The Limits of Community-Based Theatre:
    Performance and HIV Prevention in Tanzania', *The Drama Review* 54:1
    (T205), (Winter 2010), New York and Cambridge, MA: New York University
    and Massachusetts Institute of Technology.

## Chapter 1   HIV Prevention as Community-Based Theatre

1. My friend and colleague Stephen Ndibalema, who worked with me during
   my fieldwork in Kagera in 2006, lived in Bukoba in 1987. In those days it
   seemed that people went to a funeral more than once a day, he told me and
   went on: 'If close relatives die, you normally shave your head and mourn
   for 40 days. But people just couldn't shave after a while. Their heads were
   already naked. People couldn't even work because of all the funerals. So
   people started to change the traditions: they stopped shaving and stopped
   wearing casual dresses on funerals (which is a custom since it shows that you
   are not enjoying the occasion but that you are concerned). People started to
   wear nice clothes. People also came with plastic bags. In connection to that
   a saying became established: "When did you receive the news?" (i.e., about
   someone dying, whose funeral you had to attend without notice, which

is why the plastic bag became the most convenient baggage). The plastic bag was therefore called *wabimanya maki*, meaning "when did you get the news?".'

2. For more information about the possible origin of the HIV virus, see: http://www.avert.org/origin-aids-hiv.htm (accessed 15 April 2010).

3. AIDS is the new 'great imitator', according to Sabin (1987). This follows upon the old characterization of syphilis as a great imitator of other diseases.

4. This relates especially to poor outcomes for malaria, which are often caused by rural people arriving too late with their children to dispensaries after lengthy journeys, not seldom by foot. But the long distances and the scarce logistical means will also have an impact on the distribution of anti-retroviral medicines for a long time to come.

5. In the movie *Traffic*, Michael Douglas said something interesting as he depicted an American politician who steps down as head of the so-called war on drugs, while agonizing over his son's cocaine addiction: 'How can you wage war on your own family?'

6. The lack of local political commitment was recently corroborated in interviews with a big organization like UNAIDS (interview with programme associate Henry Meena in Dar es Salaam, 21 May 2007) as well as the smaller Forum for Grassroots Organizations in Tanzania (FOGOTA; interview with Secretary General Emmanuel Kazungu in Dar es Salaam, 25 May 2007).

7. In 25 years AIDS is estimated to have killed about 25 million people and infected 65 million; thus nearly 40 million are currently living with the virus. UNAIDS/WHO, 'Report on the Global AIDS Epidemic', Geneva, available at: http://www.unaids.org (accessed May 2006). As Nugent points out (with reference to R. Shell, 'Halfway to the Holocaust: The Economic, Demographic, and Social Implications of the AIDS Pandemic to the year 2010 in the Southern African Region', in R. Shell et al., eds, *HIV/AIDS: A Threat to the African Renaissance* (Johannesburg: Konrad Adenauer Stiftung, 2000), p. 10), 'It is estimated that by 2010, AIDS will have killed more people than all of the previous global pandemics – including the Black Death, smallpox in the sixteenth century and the devastating 1917/19 influenza outbreak – combined' (P. Nugent, *Africa since Independence: A Comparative History* (New York: Palgrave Macmillan, 2004), pp. 357–8).

8. Tears do not transmit the virus, but have a certain viral load, just like other bodily fluids. See H. Jackson, *AIDS Africa: Continent in Crisis*. (Harare: SAfAIDS, 2002).

9. Needless to say, monetary and clinical approaches to AIDS are necessary complements to preventive measures through human resources. It is just that money and pills have for long overshadowed cultural factors in the expertise of the epidemic. Anti-retroviral medicines have been distributed *en masse* by WHO in a global scheme called '3 in 5' – alluding to the ambition to reach three million people in five years – but they keep missing their goals even in areas for which they have secured funding and medical supplies. The incidence rates simply exceed the logistical possibilities of distributing medicine in many countries.

10. Writing from a female perspective, of course, involves certain ethical risks, not only about being taken as a white man who wants to save brown women

from brown men, as G. C. Spivak puts it ('Can the Subaltern Speak?', in Cary Nelson and Lawrence Grossberg, eds, *Marxism and the Interpretation of Culture* (Urbana: University of Illinois Press, 1988), pp. 271–313), but also due to the epistemological risk of alienating men in an epidemic which is ultimately about establishing gender-balanced negotiations and solutions. Nonetheless, according to statistical data, general research, my own performance analyses, focus-group discussions, and interviews (see below), it is undeniable that the most critical risk factors and perilous experiences of the epidemic are female.

11. M. Pompêo Nogueira, 'Theatre for Development: An Overview', *Research in Drama Education*, 7, 1 (2002); D. Kerr, *African Popular Theatre: From Pre-colonial Times to the Present Day* (Nairobi: East African Educational Publishers, 1995); J. Bakari and G. Materego, *Sanaa kwa Maendeleo: Stadi, Mbinu na Mazoezi* (Dar es Salaam: Amana Publishers, 1995); Z. Mda, *When People Play People* (London: ZED Books Ltd, 1993); P. Mlama, *Culture and Development* (Uppsala: Nordiska Afrikainstitutet, 1991); C. Kamlongera, *Theatre for Development in Africa with Case Studies from Malawi and Zambia* (Bonn: German Foundation for International Development, 1989); R. Kidd, *From People's Theatre for Revolution to Popular Theatre for Reconstruction: Diary of a Zimbabwean Workshop* (The Hague/Toronto: CESO, 1984a), to mention but a few.

12. D. Kerr, 'Art as Tool, Weapon or Shield? Arts for Development Seminar, Harare', in Biodun Jeyifo, ed., *Modern African Drama* (New York: W. W. Norton, 2002); D. Byam, *Community in Motion: Theatre for Development in Africa* (Westport, CT: Bergin and Garvey, 1999); J. Plastow, *African Theatre and Politics: The Evolution of Theatre in Ethiopia, Tanzania and Zimbabwe. A Comparative Study* (Amsterdam: Editions Rodopi, B.V., 1996).

13. O. Abah, 'Creativity, Participation and Change in Theatre for Development Practice', in Francis Harding, ed., *The Performance Arts in Africa: A Reader* (New York and London: Routledge, 2002), pp. 158–73.

14. M. Frank, *AIDS Education through Theatre: Case Studies from Uganda* (Bayreuth: Bayreuth African Studies, 1995).

15. R. Mabala et. al., *Participatory Action Research on HIV/AIDS through a Popular Theatre Approach in Tanzania* (Unicef: Evaluation and Programme Planning, 2002); M. Klink, 'Theatre for Development', in Hands On! A Manual for Working with Youth on SRH (GTZ: 2000), available at: http://www2. unescobkk.org/hivaids/FullTextDB/aspUploadFiles/HandsOnPublikation.pdf (accessed 28 October 2006).

16. L. Bourgault, *Playing for Life: Performance in Africa in the Age of AIDS* (Durham, NC: Carolina Academic Press, 2003).

17. B. Crow and M. Etherton, 'Popular Drama and Popular Analysis in Africa', in R. Kidd and N. Colletta, eds, *Tradition for Development: Indigenous Structures and Folk Media in Non-formal Education* (Bonn: German Foundation for International Development, 1982).

18. Kidd, 'From People's Theatre'; P. Freire, *Pedagogy of the Oppressed* (New York: Herder & Herder, 1970).

19. O. Abah and M. Etherton, 'The Samaru Projects: Street Theatre in Northern Nigeria', *Theatre Research International*, 7 (1983), pp. 222–34; O. Abah and S. Balewa, *The Bomo Project* (Zaria, Nigeria: English Department, Ahmadu Bello

University, 1982); A. Boal, *Theatre of the Oppressed*, trans. Charles A. and Maria-Odilia Leal McBride (London: Pluto Press, 1979).

20. Mda, *When People Play People*; Byam, *Community in Motion*, ch. 3; P. Mlama, *Culture and Development*, chs 4–5; F. P. Nyoni, *Conformity and Change: Tanzanian Rural Theatre and Socio-political Changes* (doctoral dissertation, University of Leeds, 1998).

21. Paulo Freire is one of the most influential educationalists in the twentieth century, especially for his theories on progressive practice for impoverished and oppressed people in Latin America, Africa, and Asia. Freire's *Pedagogy of the Oppressed* (1970) inspired fellow Brazilian Augusto Boal to develop the methods for his so-called 'theatre of the oppressed'.

22. The project was lead by Penina Mlama, Amandina Lihamba and Eberhard Chambulikazi from The Fine and Performing Arts Department at The University of Dar es Salaam, Tanzania, who are among the chief innovators of the TFD community process (for a detailed description on the project, see Mlama 1991, ch. 7).

23. In a Tanzanian village called Ijumbe in 2004, it was remarkable to see almost all male spectators, after enjoying an *ngoma* (dance), turn around and go back to their market stands as they heard the opening stanza of a choir on AIDS.

24. Frank, *AIDS Education through Theatre*; G. Kwesigabo, *Trends of HIV Infection in the Kagera Region of Tanzania* (Umeå University Medical Dissertations, New Series No. 710, 2001); B. Jordan-Harder, 'Thirteen Years of HIV-1 Sentinel Surveillance and Indicators for Behavioural Change Suggest Impact of Programme Activities in south-west Tanzania', *AIDS*, 18 (2004): 287–94.

25. Femi Osofisan (in R. Boon and J. Plastow, eds, *Theatre Matters: Performance and Culture on the World Stage* (Cambridge: Cambridge University Press, 1998), pp. 11–35) considers students and other educated cohorts the most important target groups for radical theatre, rather than the proletariat favoured by, e.g., Ngugi wa Thiong'o and most other developmental theatre artists and groups in Africa. There are countless school projects involving theatre against AIDS in Africa, but they are mostly temporary and lack financial, administrative and moral support. It is not uncommon that teachers have sex with students, while being reluctant towards sexual and reproductive schooling due to its encouragement of promiscuous lifestyles. For country-specific views on theatre as education, see also S. Lange, *Managing Modernity: Gender, State, and Nation in the Popular Drama of Dar es Salaam, Tanzania* (University of Bergen: Department of Social Anthropology, 2002); L. Edmondson, 'National Erotica: The Politics of "Traditional" Dance in Tanzania', *Drama Review*, 45:1/T 169 (2001): 153–70; T. Riccio, 'Tanzanian Theatre: From Marx to the Marketplace', *Drama Review*, 45:1/T 169 (2001): 128–52; Hatar, *Theatising AIDS for Paralegal Organisations*.

26. The artistic extension workers were Amandina Lihamba, Penina Mlama, and Eberhard Chambulikazi, all from the University of Dar es Salaam, Tanzania.

27. Besides the numerous plays, a few interesting films have also depicted sugar daddies, such as the Tanzanian film *Duara* (2003), collectively written by students at the Fine and Performing Arts Department, University of Dar es Salaam, and directed by Richard Ndunguru.

## Chapter 2    The Performativity of Community-Based Theatre

1.  This is obviously a qualified truth; see, for instance, Turner's remarks about British interference among the Ndembu in connection with the Ihamba cult (Turner 1967: 359–93; esp. 374).

2.  This also concerned the Ndembu to a certain extent. Just to give one example, Turner writes that he came upon a Ndembu man in the Copperbelt mining town of Chingola who asserted that 'he was never going back to village life' (Turner 1967: 391). For an updated account on the life of the Lunda-Ndembu, see Pritchett (2001).

3.  For further discussion of gendered aspects of Turner's ethnography, see the essay by Andrew Wegley in Franko (2006).

4.  There are some traditional medicines that mitigate the effect of AIDS-related opportunistic infections and diseases. Hence, medicine is certainly an area where traditional knowledge should be combined with modern biomedicine (for more on this, see 'Collaboration with traditional healers in HIV/AIDS prevention and care in sub-Saharan Africa' (UNAIDS 2000)). Most people in Africa still consult traditional rather than modern doctors. In light of this fact and the widespread lack of anti-retroviral medicines, people's hesitation about taking a HIV-test is quite logical. Reyonolds Whyte writes: 'In 1995, many people spoke of the need to have AIDS testing in Bunyole [Uganda]. I suspect that this idea is attractive as a way of resolving the uncertainty about others. However, it is not clear that worried people would choose to resolve the uncertainty about themselves by seeking a test – at least not without persuasion and counselling. It is better not to know for sure that you are doomed' (1997: 214).

5.  Forum theatre is an interactive form of performance, in which spectators – or 'spect-actors' – can intervene both verbally and physically in critical scenes and suggest alternative solutions. It was invented by the Brazilian theatre pedagogue Augusto Boal in the 1960s and has had a great influence on popular theatre in Africa due to its adaptability to local modes of storytelling, dialogue, and improvisation.

6.  I will not comment on Jacques Derrida's or anyone else's criticism of Austin's speech act theory here, but simply suggest that readers look up a most clarifying arbitration of the arguments involved in Stanley Cavell's *A Pitch of Philosophy: Autobiographical Exercises* (1996: ch. 2). Nor will I comment on Austin's exclusion of theatre from his reasoning in *How to Do Things with Words*, which I believe was made for the sake of philosophical clarity in his Harvard lectures; I am also confident that the above-mentioned performance in the South African school workshop would have appealed to Austin to such an extent that he would have found it impossible to exclude it as a philosophically pertinent example due to its, at once, ordinary *and* ceremonial case of performative speech.

7.  I have criticized both the sociological and anthropological stereotypology of theatre elsewhere (Johansson 2006; 2002).

8.  See the six conventions for an explicit performative to take effect (Austin 1962: 14–15; also Austin 1979: 237).

9. It should be clear that Kerr uses the word 'theatre' in a very wide sense, namely 'to cover drama, many forms of ritual, dance, and other performing arts such as acrobatics, mime and semi-dramatized narratives' (Kerr 1995: 1).

10. To inform, warn, and persuade someone typify certain kinds of Austinian speech acts, namely, respectively, locutionary acts (simply by uttering something meaningful, such as the term 'AIDS' in a site where it is rarely enunciated), illocutionary acts (e.g., alerting people of a danger), and perlocutionary acts (by convincing people of a hazard).

11. One of the most valuable qualities of Louise Bourgault's book *Playing for Life* (2004) is its many examples of chants and songs (ch. 6) that have shaped the public opinion of some African countries when it comes to AIDS. One of these songs is indeed Philly Luutaya's *Alone* (Bourgault 2004: 164).

12. An individual's blood *serum* converts after exposure to the virus, from HIV antibody negative to antibody positive. This conversion can be quantified and thus measured in terms of, e.g., the need to set dosage in anti-retroviral medicine.

13. For the use of metaphors on AIDS in the West, see Sontag 1988.

14. It is worth pointing out that the pre-colonial performances called *mashindano* in East Africa took place in communal events that functioned as competitions (Gunderson and Barz 2000).

## Chapter 3 The Social Drama of Backstage Discourse and Performance

1. I had the privilege of working with Stephen Ndibalema, a teacher at The Fine and Performing Arts Department, University of Dar es Salaam, during my fieldworks in Kagera 2006. Stephen grew up in Kagera and is an artistic as well as academic expert on the region's performance traditions. In 2004 I worked with Priscus Kainunula, who works with the non-governmental organization Humuuliza, one of the most important civil services for orphans in Kagera. When I visited Ilemera for the first time in 2003, John B. Joseph, programme advisor for Swissaid in Muleba, accompanied me. All three are trilingual, fluent in the local language Ruhaya, the national language Kiswahili and English.

2. In March 2003, the Clinton Foundation HIV/AIDS Initiative (CHAI) partnered with the Government of Tanzania, the Harvard AIDS Institute, and PharmAccess, and worked with a multi-sectored team comprised of the Ministry of Health, the Tanzania Commission for AIDS, cabinet agencies, Muhimbili University, local NGOs, and others to develop a business plan for providing comprehensive care and treatment to Tanzanians living with HIV/AIDS. However, it took a couple of years to allocate the medicine to many of the regional and district hospitals in Tanzania. In a regionalized initiative, CHAI was allocated to the southern regions of Mtwara and Lindi (*UNGASS Country Progress Report: Tanzania Mainland* (2008), Dar es Salaam: Tanzania Commission for AIDS, p. 34).

3. *Kagera Region: Socio-Economic Profile* (Dar es Salaam: National Bureau of Statistics (NBS)/Kagera Regional Commissioner's Office, August 2003), ix.

4.  Vanessa von Struensee writes: 'Although Tanzania's Law of Marriage Act, 1971, (LMA) recognizes marriage as a partnership and declares that any property acquired during the existence of a marriage is joint matrimonial property, the LMA does not apply to inheritance and does not supersede customary law. Thus, the discriminatory rules continue to apply to succession matters to the detriment of widows. Worse still is the customary practice governed by Rule 62, of wife inheritance, where a widow is required to marry a male relative of her dead spouse. If she agrees, she can remain there as a wife, but with no claim or control over the land. Women succumb to widow inheritance under duress where the alternative is destitution.' ('Widows, AIDS, Health, and Human Rights in Africa', http://www.crisisstates.com/download/forum/HIV/901widowsaids.pdf, pp. 25–6, 2005. Last visited in April 2007. This can be compared with the governmental legislation of the Married Women's Property Act in 1882 in the United Kingdom, under which married women had the same rights over their property as unmarried women and allowed a married woman to retain ownership of property which she might have received as a gift from a parent. In 1893 the Act was broadened, as married women were given full legal control of all the property of every kind which they owned at marriage or that they acquired after marriage, either by inheritance or by their own earnings. Interestingly, Elin Diamond refers to the Married Women's Property Act in her analysis of Ibsen's *Hedda Gabler*, see 'The Violence of "We": Politicizing Identification', in Janelle G. Reinelt and Joseph R. Roach (eds.), *Critical Theory and Performance* (Ann Arbor: The University of Michigan Press, 1992), pp. 390–412.

5.  Japhet Killewo, *Epidemiology towards the control of HIV infection in Tanzania with special reference to the Kagera region* (Umeå: Umeå University, Department of Epidemiology and Public Health, 1994).

6.  Transactional sex is not, as Western prostition may be, a full-time occupation but more of a temporary, or more or less regular, opportunity to make ends meet, mainly for destitute women. Transactional sex mostly involve a cash deal but often other kinds of gifts as well.

7   Suicide is, of course, also an option and an often ventilated one. It is as if this fatalistic taboo is less unmentionable than the syndrome that causes it. To show a suicide attempt in performance is unusual, though. One exception took place in a performance by a theatre group in Bukoba town, where a disinherited widow tried to hang herself but gets saved by a neighbour at the last second. About a hundred noisy marketplace spectators quieted down in a moment, as if seeing something they had merely heard – or possibly thought – of before, if not experienced surreptitiously.

8.  The islands are notorious for their HIV/AIDS prevalence. In 1997, several years after the epidemic peaked in Uganda and Tanzania, a Lake Victoria fishing community was studied by Pickering and Okongo et al., who found that '[i]ts men had on average one new sexual partner every twelve days' (quoted in Iliffe *The African AIDS Epidemic: A History*, pp. 24, 165). It is also worth pointing out that when I asked the Ilemera group what they consider to be the major risk factors of HIV/AIDS in their (Muleba) district (cf. Questionnaire/Appendix II), they respond: 'Sexual behaviour on the islands' (group interview in Ilemera, 3 August 2006.) There are 18 islands within the bounds of Muleba District in Lake Victoria.

9. An alternative and more contemporaneous scenario is mentioned here. When young diseased women have made money on the islands by transactional sex, they can afford going back to the mainland and establishing a lifestyle using ARV therapy (group interview in Ilemera, 3 August 2006.) This statement seems to suggest that maintaining an ARV regimen requires a certain amount of money, which is of course true in terms of transport and other side-costs in connection to hospital visits. Eventually regions like Kagera and countries like Tanzania will also have to carry all or parts of the cost of the medicine.

10. David Kerr, *African Popular Theatre: From Pre-Colonial Times to the Present Day* (Nairobi: East African Educational Publishers, 1995), p. 160.

11. 'There is overwhelming evidence about the efficacy and effectiveness of condoms when used correctly and consistently in the prevention of HIV transmission. Good quality condoms shall be produced and made easily available and affordable. The private sector shall be encouraged to produce and market good quality condoms so that they are easily accessible in urban and rural areas' (*National Policy on HIV/AIDS*, sec. 5.10, 2001).

12. It is a well-known fact that all major faith-based organizations in Tanzania – including not only Catholics but also Lutherans, Anglicans, and Muslims – are officially opposed to the promotion, distribution, and use of condoms. In a joint statement at a convention in Dar es Salaam in 2002, 70 representatives from the major religions made it clear that they discourage their followers from using condoms due to the fact that all holy books are opposed to the use of condoms (Clerics' Condom Stand At Odds With National Policy in *UN Integrated Regional Information Networks – March 18, 2002*; http://www. aegis.com/news/irin/2002/Ir020305.html (last accessed 15 August 2007).

13. Nyanje, P. 'HIV/Aids Debate Hots Up', *The Guardian in Dar es Salaam* (31 July 2002); for an online version, see *UN Integrated Regional Information Networks – August 20, 2002*: http://www.aegis.com/news/IRIN/2002/IR020806.html (last accessed 15 August 2007).

14. For further reading on the moral implications of allowing versus doing harm, see, for instance, Philippa Foot, 'Morality, Action and Outcome', in Ted Honderich, ed., *Morality and Objectivity* (London: Routledge & Kegan Paul, 1985), and Warren S. Quinn, 'Actions, Intentions, and Consequences: The Doctrine of Doing and Allowing', in A. Norcross and B. Steinbock, eds, *Killing and Letting Die*, 2nd edn (New York: Fordham University Press, 1994). For more specific reading on how ideology comes in between national (South African) attitudes on AIDS and people's need for protection, see Catherine Campbell,'*Letting them Die': How HIV/AIDS Programmes often Fail* (Oxford: James Currey, 2003).

15. In the districts of Masasi and Mangaka of Mtwara region. Apart from Margaret Malenga (2003), I have worked with Andrew Hamisi (2003 and 2004), and Delphine Njewele (2006).

16. This reasoning is, of course, inspired by Erving Goffman's notion of, and approach to, social front- and backstage performances in *The Presentation of Self in Everyday Life* (Garden City, NY: Doubleday; Anchor Books, 1959), see esp. p. 112.

17. I am using most of the research methods that Ann Bowling defines in health studies: 'Qualitative research describes in words rather than numbers the

qualities of social phenomena through observation (direct and unobtrusive or participative and reactive), unstructured interviews (or 'exploratory', 'in-depth', 'free-style' interviews, usually tape recorded and then transcribed before analysis), diary methods, life histories (biography), group interviews and focus group techniques, analysis of historical and contemporary records, documents and cultural products (e.g. media and literature).' *Research Methods in Health: Investigating Health and Health Services* (Maidenhead: Open University Press, 2004), p. 352.

18. Statistical gender discrepancies are found in a number of reports in Tanzania (see 'HIV/AIDS/STI Surveillance Report: January–October 2004', United Republic of Tanzania: Ministry of Health/National AIDS Control Programme, Report No. 19, October 2005) as well as in sub-Saharan Africa in general ('Report on the Global AIDS Epidemic', December 2006). Hence, women are more exposed to HIV and, in the words of a Ugandan representative at the fifteenth International AIDS Conference in Bangkok in 2004, it is statistically more dangerous to be a housewife than a soldier in Africa.

19. The statistics for 2006 reads as follows in the Ilemera ward, where the community centre in question deploys extension workers: Among 86 people living with HIV/AIDS (PLWHA) 13 were male and 73 female. These numbers – which are not scientifically validated but indicative of local incidence and prevalence trends – point to a greater willingness among females to seek or be recruited for medical attention and also a great number of absent men in general. But the statistics are also indicative of the above-mentioned gender discrepancies.

20. 'HIV/AIDS/STI Surveillance Report: January–October 2004', United Republic of Tanzania: Ministry of Health/National AIDS Control Programme, Report No. 19, October 2005), p. 2.

21. Gideon Kwesigabo, *Trends of HIV infection in the Kagera Region of Tanzania 1987–2000* (Umeå University Medical Dissertations, New Series No. 710, 2001).

22. 'HIV/AIDS/STI Surveillance Report: January–October 2004', United Republic of Tanzania: Ministry of Health/National AIDS Control Programme, Report No. 19, October 2005), pp. 26–7. Hanson (2007: 7) confirms these figures with reference to Kwesigabo. 1987 Muleba had an estimated prevalence rate of 10 per cent, in 1996 it had declined to 7 per cent and 1999 it was down to 4 per cent.

23. Judith Narrow (2003): unpublished document.

24. *Vipi mambo* is a fashionable, contemporary, and urban way of greeting a peer. Tanzania is a country where greeting ceremonials have been, and in many places still are, considered as an important indicator of respect and social status. *Mambo* derives from *jambo*, as in *Hujambo!*, which roughly means 'What is your news?', which is always followed by a positive response such as *Nzuri sana*, 'Just fine' or something like it. (A variant of this is mentioned in the following paragraph, namely *vipi kaka* [brother].) It is not uncommon that young people, especially in rural areas, greet elders with the word *Shikamuu!*, to which the elder responds *Marahaba!* The latter is a greeting ceremonial from the early era of Arabic slavery in the fourteenth and fifteenth centuries, with quite controversial political roots. However, for a young women to address an old man with any other phrase than *Shikamuu!*

would be considered as disgraceful just ten years ago, before the urbanization of rural sociolects in Tanzania.

25. This was said by Dr Alex Coutinho from the Ugandan The AIDS Support
Organization (TASO) during a speech at SIDA in Stockholm, Sweden,
3 August 2007: http://www.youtube.com/watch?v=HX8xkdJ47YY (accessed
19 April 2010).

26. The component called 'community analysis' in some applied theatre projects
can, for instance, make use of more thorough and hands-on modes of action
research, such as organized fieldwork with focus group discussions and
interviews. This may sound too academic but it can, I believe, be used in a
quite simple and yet trustworthy and conscientious way by taking in shared
and intimate stories from fellow community residents and thereby enhance
their respect. (Of course such initiatives presuppose a more serious political
and civil backing from project stakeholders, but this is, I believe, a premise
to *any* qualitative improvement of CBT against AIDS.) A more methodical
and thorough use of action research would also provide an entry point to
a more differentiated analysis of male and female experiences of HIV/AIDS.
It is worth repeating that the gender factors, more than any other, could be
made much more explicit in most of the community performances I have
seen.

27. During our visit in July 2003, we saw pamphlets and other text material from
UNICEF on some bookshelves in the youth centre.

## Chapter 4   A Deadly Paradox: Assessing the Success/Failure of Community-Based Theatre against AIDS

1. It is by now clear that sub-Saharan Africa will not fulfil the millennium goals
set for 2015 (for a discussion of this, see Easterly 2007).

2. An alternative vocabulary for the mobile and containing features of CBT
would be to use Robert Putnam's (2000) terms of 'bonding' and 'bridging'
social capital. The latter concept has already been put to the test in an
important social study on the limits of HIV prevention work in South Africa
by Campbell (2003). The task of bridging communal divisions is a greater
and more significant challenge than bonding individual groups.

3. It is important not to tap into defeatist fear mongering about 'AIDS Africa'.
Irobi (2006: 32) asserts that the 'overall tragic prognosis is that these children
are destined to die unless world governments, drug companies, politicians
in both the rich Western countries and the impoverished African countries
can work out a pragmatic programme for treating the infected, particularly the AIDS orphans, for whom the beginning of life has now become
the commencement of an agonizing death sentence'. It is true that many
AIDS orphans are left without care, but at least as many are taken care of
by grandparents, who have taken on an overwhelming and unprecedented
responsibility. In all fairness, it should also be said that international donors
have put quite heavy emphasis on orphan care. Painting broad and general-
izing strokes of catastrophe only serves to enhance Western caricatures of
Africa. Among the many elderly guarantors I have met in Africa, a woman
called Beatrice in Nairobi, Kenya, stands out as a special person. She lives in

the Mathare slum in Nairobi and takes care of about 40 grandchildren after all of her own eight children perished in AIDS-related diseases. She is now doing all right by participating in a sustainable micro-finance programme set up by the organization Jamii Bora.

4. For a sociological study on women working as housemaids in Tanzania, see Heggenhougen and Lugalla (2005: ch. 13).

5. The religious intervention is indicative of the Christian interest organization behind the theatre group, the conservative World Vision. If the priest is inquiring about love according to the creed of World Vision, it is certainly a matter of faithful bonds within monogamous relationships. If the person is not yet married, she or he should abstain from sex until marriage. However, in reality it is much more likely that the love in question is challenged by materialistic and financial constraints and incentives (for an interesting study on the commodification of relationships in Tanzania, see Setel 1999).

6. M. Banham, ed., *A History of Theatre in Africa* (Cambridge: Cambridge University Press, 2004), p. 305.

7. See: http://www.entersoftsystems.com/tacaids/documents/NMSF%20% 202008%20-2012.pdf (last visited in August 2009).

8. In a significant report for UNESCO, Hatar (2001) cracks the myth on performing arts as naturally integrated in Tanzanian society by showing what little support they have received in the educational system since independence.

9. Kerr makes the observation of the constant risk of self-blame in Theatre for Development, where poverty stricken theatre workers tend to fall into the paradoxical stance of 'scapegoating the poor' (Kerr 1995: 160).

10. *FHI/UNAIDS Best Practices in HIV/AIDS Prevention Collection* (2001), ed. Bunmi Makinwa and Mary O'Grady: http://www.fhi.org/NR/rdonlyres/e3hmq5w4 o542tmtlhi66rtwqijhfqqzgaspcwkc55f327e6dvdc5a2d5zwjdbdhhl7mgw6 bprtmhip/FHIUNAIDSBestPracticesreduxenhv.pdf (accessed 9 April 2010).

11. There is a prolific and long-term project called Tuseme ('Let Us Speak Out' in Swahili), which is implemented for girls in secondary schools and based on the principles of Theatre for Development. It has yet to be properly evaluated, but exemplifies both qualitative and quantitative qualities in the application of social theatre. CBT is closely related to theatre activities like Tuseme, but it also takes on the precarious challenge of mobilizing out-of-school youth, since they represent a majority in their age brackets and are likely to be more closely associated with the most susceptible youth in the pandemic.

# Bibliography

Abah, Oga S. (2002) 'Creativity, participation and change in Theatre for Development practice', in Francis Harding, ed., *The Performance Arts in Africa: A Reader*. New York and London: Routledge, pp. 158–73.

Abah, O. and Balewa, S. (1982) *The Bomo Project*. Zaria, Nigeria: English Department, Ahmadu Bello University.

Abah, O. and Etherton, M. (1983) 'The Samaru Projects: Street Theatre in Northern Nigeria', *Theatre Research International*, 7.

Ahlberg, B. M., et.al. (1997) 'Male Circumcision: Meaning, Organisation, Practice and Implications for Transmission and Prevention', *African Sociological Review*, 1:1: 66–81.

Ajzen, I. (1980) *Understanding the Attitudes and Predicting Social Behaviour*. Englewood Cliffs, NJ: Prentice-Hall.

Appleton, J. (2000) '"At my age I should be sitting under that tree": The Impact of AIDS on Tanzanian Lakeshore Communities', *Gender and Development*, 8:2.

Arnfred, S., ed. (2004) *Re-Thinking Sexualities in Africa*. Uppsala: Almqvist & Wiksell.

Austin, J. L. (1979) *Philosophical Papers*. Oxford: Clarendon Press.

Austin, J. L. (1962) *How to Do Things with Words*. Oxford: Clarendon Press.

Bakari, J. and Materego, G. (1995) *Sanaa kwa Maendeleo: Stadi, Mbinu na Mazoezi*. Dar es Salaam: Amana Publishers.

Banham, M., ed. (2004) *A History of Theatre in Africa*. Cambridge: Cambridge University Press.

Barba, E. (1986) *The Floating Islands*. New York: PAJ Publications.

Barnett, T. and Blaikie, P. M. (1992) *AIDS in Africa: Its Present and Future Impact*. London: Belhaven Press.

Barnett, T. and Whiteside, A. (2002) *AIDS in the 21st Century: Disease and Globalisation*. Basingstoke: Palgrave Macmillan.

Barongo, G. (1998) *The Function of Omutoro Dance is More for the Praising of Heroes than for Instruction*, BA Dissertation, University of Dar Es Salaam.

Barthes, R. (1977) *Image Music Text*. London: Fontana Press.

Bell, C. (1997) *Ritual: Perspectives and Dimensions*. New York and Oxford: Oxford University Press.

Biodun, J., ed. (2002) *Modern African Drama*. New York: W. W. Norton.

Bloch, M. (1992) *Prey into Hunter: The Politics of Religious Experience*. Cambridge: Cambridge University Press.

Boal, A. (1979) *Theatre of the Oppressed*, trans. Charles A. and Maria-Odilia Leal McBride. London: Pluto Press.

Boon, R. and Plastow, J. eds (1998) *Theatre Matters: Performance and Culture on the World Stage*. Cambridge: Cambridge University Press.

Bourgault, L. (2003) *Playing for Life: Performance in Africa in the Age of AIDS*. Durham, NC: Carolina Academic Press.

Bowling, A. (2004) *Research Methods in Health: Investigating Health and Health Services*. New York: Open University Press.

Butler, J. (1997) *Excitable Speech*. London and New York: Routledge.

Byam, D. L. (1999) *Community in Motion: Theatre for Development in Africa*. London: Bergin & Garvey.

Bynum, Caroline Walker (1984) 'Women's Stories, Women's Symbols: A Critique of Victor Turner's Theory of Liminality', in R. L. Moore and F. E. Reynolds, eds, *Anthropology and the Study of Religion*. Chicago: Center for the Scientific Study of Religion.

Campbell, C. (2003) *'Letting Them Die': How HIV/AIDS Prevention Programmes often Fail*. Oxford: James Currey.

Cavell, S. (1994) *A Pitch of Philosophy: Autobiographical Exercises*. Cambridge, MA: Harvard University Press.

Clifford, J. (1986) 'On Ethnographic Allegory', in J, Clifford and G. E. Marcus, eds, *Writing Culture: Experiments in Contemporary Anthropology*. Berkeley and Los Angeles: University of California Press.

Cohen-Cruz, J. (1999) 'Practice & Policy in Theatre & Development', in M. Banham, J. Gibbs, and F. Osofisan, eds, *African Theatre in Development*. Oxford: James Currey.

Conner, M. and Norman, P. (1996) *Predicting Health Behavior: Search and Practice with Social Cognition Models*. Buckingham: Open University Press.

Coutinho, A. (2007) The AIDS Support Organization (TASO), speech at SIDA in Stockholm, Sweden, 3 August 2007. See http://www.youtube.com/watch?vHX8xkdJ47YY (accessed 19 April 2010).

Crow, B. and Etherton, M. (1982) 'Popular Drama and Popular Analysis in Africa', in R. Kidd and N. Colletta, eds, *Tradition for Development: Indigenous Structures and Folk Media in Non-Formal Education*. Bonn: German Foundation for International Development.

Dilger, H. (2002) 'Silences and Rumours in Discourses on AIDS in Tanzania. On the Meaning of Culture in the Growing Epidemic'. Paper presented at the conference 'Language, Literature and the Discourse of HIV/AIDS in Africa' at the University of Botswana, 24–28 June 2002.

Dilger, H. (2001) 'AIDS in Africa: Broadening the Perspectives on Research and Policy-Making', *Afrika spectrum*, 36:1.

Easterly, W. (2007) 'How the Millenium Development Goals are Unfair to Africa', see: http://www.brookings.edu/~/media/Files/rc/papers/2007/11_poverty_easterly/11_poverty_easterly.pdf (accessed 1 May 2010).

Edmondson, L. (2001) 'National Erotica: The Politics of "Traditional" Dance in Tanzania', *The Drama Review*, 45:1 (T 169): 153–70.

Eyoh, Ansel (1986) 'Hammocks and Bridges'. Workshop on Theatre for Integrated Rural Development. Yaoundé: University of Yaoundé.

Fanon, F. (1968) *The Wretched of the Earth*. New York: Grove Press.

Feldhendler, Daniel (1994) 'Augusto Boal and Jacob L. Moreno: Theatre and Therapy', in M. Schutzman and J. Cohen-Cruz, eds, *Playing Boal: Theatre, Activism, Therapy*. London and New York: Routledge, pp. 87–109.

Foreman, Martin, ed. (1999) *AIDS and Men: Taking Risks or Taking Responsibility?* London: Panos/Zed Books.

Frank, Marion (1995) *AIDS Education through Theatre: Case Studies from Uganda*, doctoral dissertation. Bayreuth: Bayreuth African Studies.

Franko, M., ed. (2006) *Ritual and Event: Interdisciplinary Perspectives*. London and New York: Routledge.

Freire, P. (1970) *Pedagogy of the Oppressed*. New York: Herder & Herder.

Freudenthal, S. (2002) 'A Review of Social Science Research on Hiv/Aids'. Paper prepared for Swedish International Development and Cooperation Agency (SIDA).

Gausset, Q. (2001) 'AIDS and Cultural Practices in Africa: The Case of the Tonga (Zambia)', *Social Science and Medicine*, 52.

Gerholm, T. (1988) 'On Ritual: A Postmodernist View', *Ethnos*, 53. Stockholm: Almqvist & Wiksell International.

Giddens, A. (1984) *The Constitution of Society: Outline of the Theory of Structuration*. Cambridge: Polity Press.

Gilbert, H. and Tompkins, J., eds (1996) *Post-Colonial Drama: Theory, Practice, Politics*. London and New York: Routledge.

Goffman, E. (1974) *Frame Analysis: An Essay on the Organization of Experience*. Cambridge, MA: Harvard University Press.

Goffman, E. (1959) *The Presentation of Self in Everyday Life*. Garden City, NY: Doubleday; Anchor Books.

Görgen, R., ed. (2002) *Hands On!: A Manual for Working with Youth on SRH*, GTZ, see: http://www2.unescobkk.org/hivaids/FullTextDB/aspUploadFiles/HandsOnPublikation.pdf (accessed 2 May 2010).

Green, A. E. (1995) 'Ritual', entry in *The Cambridge Guide to Theatre*. Cambridge: Cambridge University Press.

Grimes, R. L. (2000) *Deeply into the Bone: Re-Inventing Rites of Passage*. Berkeley: University of California Press.

Gunderson, F. and Barz, G. F. (2000) *Mashindano! Competitive Music Performance in East Africa*. Dar es Salaam: Mkuki na Nyota Publishers.

Hansson, S. (2007) *Control of HIV and other Sexually Transmitted Infections: Studies in Tanzania and Zambia*. Stockholm: diss. at Division of International Health, Karolinska Institutet.

Harding, F. (ed.) (2002) *The Performance Arts in Africa: A Reader*. New York and London: Routledge.

Hatar, A. (2001) 'Theatising AIDS for Paralegal Organisations: A Report Prepared for the Friedrich Ebert Foundation'. Dar es Salaam, Tanzania.

Heggenhougen, K. and Lugalla, J., eds (2005) *Social Change and Health in Tanzania*. Dar es Salaam, Tanzania: Dar es Salaam University Press.

Holden, S., ed. (2003) *AIDS on the Agenda: Adapting Development and Humanitarian Programmes to Meet the Challenge of HIV/AIDS*. London: Oxfam Publications.

Holmdahl, B. (1988) *Människovård och människosyn: Om omvårdnad i Uppsala före år 1900*. Uppsala: Serien Uppsalas historia, Vol. VI, p. 7.

Honderich, T., ed. (1985) *Morality and Objectivity*. London: Routledge & Kegan Paul.

Iliffe, J. (2006) *The African AIDS Epidemic: A History*. Oxford: James Currey.

Iliffe, J. (2002) *East African Doctors: A History of the Modern Profession*. Kampala: Fountain Publishers.

Iliffe, J. (1995) *Africans: The Story of a Continent*. Cambridge: Cambridge University Press.

Irobi, E. (2006) 'African Youth, Performance & the HIV/AIDS Epidemic: Theatre of Necessity', in Etherton, M., ed., *African Theatre: Youth*. Oxford: James Currey.

Jackson, H. (2002) *AIDS Africa: Continent in Crisis*. Harare: SAfAIDS.

Johansson, O. (2010) 'The Limits of Community-Based Theatre: Performance and HIV Prevention in Tanzania', *The Drama Review*, 54:1 (T205), (Winter), New York and Cambridge, MA: New York University and Massachusetts Institute of Technology.

Johansson, Ola (2007a) 'The Lives and Deaths of Zakia: How AIDS Changed African Community Theatre and Vice Versa', *Theatre Research International*, 32:1.

Johansson, O. (2007b) 'Eschatological Fieldnotes: Community Theatre, AIDS, and the Fate of Informant D. in Ilemera, Tanzania', *Nordic Theatre Studies*, 13:2.

Johansson, O. (2006) 'Performative Interventions: African Community Theatre in the Age of AIDS', in *Ritual and Event: Interdisciplinary Perspectives*, ed. Mark Franko. New York and London: Routledge.

Johansson, O. (2002) 'Performative Speech in African Community Theatre on AIDS'. Paper presented at the conference 'Language, Literature and the Discourse of HIV/AIDS in Africa' at the University of Botswana, 24–28 June 2002.

Jordan-Harder, B. (2004) 'Thirteen Years of HIV-1 Sentinel Surveillance and Indicators for Behavioural Change Suggest Impact of Programme Activities in South-West Tanzania', *AIDS*, 18: 287–94.

*Kagera Region: Socio-Economic Profile* (2003). Dar es Salaam: National Bureau of Statistics (NBS)/Kagera Regional Commissioner's Office.

Kalipeni, E., et.al., eds (2004) *HIV & AIDS in Africa: Beyond Epidemiology*. Malden, MA: Blackwell Publishing.

Kamlongera, C. (1989) *Theatre for Development in Africa with Case Studies from Malawi and Zambia*. Bonn: German Foundation for International Development.

Kasfir, N., ed. (1998) *Civil Society and Democracy in Africa: Critical Perspectives*. London: Frank Cass.

Kerr, D. (2002) 'Art as Tool, Weapon or Shield? Arts for Development Seminar, Harare', in Biodun Jeyifo, ed., *Modern African Drama*. New York: W. W. Norton.

Kerr, D. (1995) *African Popular Theatre: From Pre-Colonial Times to the Present Day*. Nairobi: East African Educational Publishers.

Kidd, R. (1984a) 'From People's Theatre for Revolution to Popular Theatre for Reconstruction: Diary of a Zimbabwean Workshop'. The Hague/Toronto: CESO.

Kidd, Ross (1984b) 'Popular Theatre, Conscientization and Popular Organization'. Research paper, International Council for Adult Education. Toronto: Canada.

Kidd, R. and Colletta, N., eds (1982) *Tradition for Development: Indigenous Structures and Folk Media in Non-Formal Education*. Bonn: German Foundation for International Development.

Killewo, J. (1994) *Epidemiology towards the control of HIV infection in Tanzania with special reference to the Kagera region*. Umeå: Umeå University, Department of Epidemiology and Public Health.

Klink, M. (2000) 'Theatre for Development', in *Hands On! A Manual for Working with Youth on SRH*. GTZ, available at: http://www2.unescobkk.org/hivaids/FullTextDB/aspUploadFiles/HandsOnPublikation.pdf (accessed 28 October 2006).

Konings, E. et al. (1994) 'Sexual Behaviour Survey in a Rural Area of Northwest Tanzania', *AIDS*, 8: 997–3.

Kwesigabo, G. (2001) *Trends of HIV Infection in the Kagera Region of Tanzania*. Umeå University Medical Dissertations, New Series No. 710.

Lange, S. (2002) *Managing Modernity: Gender, State, and Nation in the Popular Drama of Dar es Salaam, Tanzania*. Doctoral dissertation, University of Bergen: Department of Social Anthropology.

Lange, S. (1995) *From Nation-Building to Popular Culture: The Modernization of Performance in Tanzania*. Report prepared for Chr. Michelsen Institute. Bergen, Norway.

Lincoln, Bruce (1991) *Emerging from the Chrysalis: Rituals of Women's Initiations*. New York: Oxford University Press.

Mabala, R., et. al. (2002) 'Participatory Action Research on HIV/AIDS through a Popular Theatre Approach in Tanzania'. UNICEF: Evaluation and Program Planning.

Mazzuki, W. M. S. (2002) 'National Response to HIV/AIDS', presentation at a UNAIDS conference, Arusha, Tanzania.

Mbembe, A. (1992) *On the Postcolony*. Berkeley and Los Angeles: University of California Press.

Mbizvo, Elizabeth. (2006) 'Essay: Theatre – A Force for Health Promotion', *The Lancet*, 368: 30–1.

Mda, Z. (1993) *When People Play People*. London: ZED Books.

Mead, George H. (1964) *Selected Writings*, ed. A. J. Reck. Chicago: University of Chicago Press.

Ministry of Health/National AIDS Control Programme (ed.) (2005 ) 'HIV/AIDS/STI Surveillance Report: January–October 2004', United Republic of Tanzania: Ministry of Health/National AIDS Control Programme, Report No. 19, October.

Mlama, P. (1991) *Culture and Development*. Uppsala: Nordiska Afrikainstitutet.

Mlelwa, H. C. (1992) *Food Shortage and Famine Problems in Masasi District: From Colonial and Post-Colonial Era (1895–1991)*. Doctoral diss. at University of Dar es Salaam.

*Mtwara: Socio-Economic Profile 1997*: 29.

Mutembei, A. K. (2001) *Poetry and AIDS in Tanzania: Changing Metaphors and Metonymies in HayaOral Traditions*. Leiden: Leiden University, Research School CNWS.

Narrow, J. (2003) Unpublished paper.

*National Policy on HIV/AIDS* (November 2001) Dodoma: The United Republic of Tanzania, Prime Minister's Office.

Nelson, C. and Grossberg, L. (eds) *Marxism and the Interpretation of Culture*. Urbana: University of Illinois Press, 1988.

Nicholson, Helen (2005) *Applied Drama: The Gift of Theatre*. Basingstoke: Palgrave Macmillan.

Norcross, A. and Steinbock, B., eds (1994) *Killing and Letting Die*. 2nd edn, New York: Fordham University Press.

Nugent, P. (2004) *Africa since Independence: A Comparative History*. New York: Palgrave Macmillan.

Nyanje, P. 'HIV/Aids Debate Hots Up', in *The Guardian in Dar es Salaam*, 31 July 2002; for an online version, see *UN Integrated Regional Information*

*Networks – August 20, 2002*: http://www.aegis.com/news/IRIN/2002/IR020806. html (last accessed 15 August 2007).

Nyoni, Frowin Paul. (2000) *Judges on Trial*. The Fine and Performing Arts Department, The University of Dar es Salaam.

Nyoni, F. P. (1998) *Conformity and Change: Tanzanian Rural Theatre and Socio-Political Changes*. Doctoral dissertation, University of Leeds.

Ormrod, J. E. (1999) *Human Learning*. Upper Saddle River, NJ: Prentice-Hall.

Plastow, J. (1996) *African Theatre and Politics: The Evolution of Theatre in Ethiopia, Tanzania and Zimbabwe. A Comparative Study*. Amsterdam: Editions Rodopi, B.V.

Pompêo Nogueira, M. (2002) 'Theatre for Development: An Overview', *Research in Drama Education*, 7:1.

Pritchett, James A. (2001) *The Lunda-Ndembu: Style, Change, and Social Transformation in South Central Africa*. Madison: University of Wisconsin Press.

Putnam, Robert. (2000) *Bowling Alone: The Collapse and Revival of American Community*. New York: Simon & Schuster.

Rappaport, R. A. (1999) *Ritual and Religion in the Making of Humanity*. Cambridge: Cambridge University Press.

Rappaport, R. A. (1968) *Pigs for the Ancestors*. New Haven, CT: Yale University Press.

Reinelt, J. G. and Roach, J. R. eds (1992) *Critical Theory and Performance*. Ann Arbor: The University of Michigan Press.

Reynolds Whyte, S. (1997) *Questioning Misfortune: The Pragmatics of Uncertainty in Eastern Uganda*. Cambridge: Cambridge University Press.

Riccio, T. (2001) 'Tanzanian Theatre: From Marx to the Marketplace', *Drama Review*, 45:1 (T 169): 128–52.

Roth Allen, Denise (2000) 'Learning the facts of Life: Past and Present Experiences in a Rural Tanzanian Community', *Africa Today*, 47:3–4.

Rubin, Don, ed. (1997) *The World Encyclopedia of Contemporary Theatre. Volume 3: Africa*. London and New York: Routledge.

Sabin, T. D. (1987) 'AIDS: The New "Great Imitator"', *The Journal of the American Geriatrics Society*, 35:5: 467–8.

Salhi, Kamal, ed. (1998) *African Theatre for Development: Art for Self-Determination*. Exeter: Intellect.

Schechner, Richard (2002) 'Ritual and Performance', in Tim Ingold, ed., *Companion Encyclopedia of Anthropology*. London and New York: Routledge.

Schechner, Richard (1988) *Performance Theory*. New York and London: Routledge.

Seppälä, P. and Koda, eds. (1998) *The Making of a Periphery*. Uppsala: Nordic Africa Institute.

Setel, Philip W. (1999) *A Plague of Paradoxes: AIDS, Culture, and Demography in Northern Tanzania*. Chicago and London: The University of Chicago Press.

Shell, R. (2000) 'Halfway to the Holocaust: The Economic, Demographic, and Social Implications of the AIDS Pandemic to the Year 2010 in the Southern African Region', in R. Shell et al., eds, *HIV/AIDS: A Threat to the African Renaissance*. Johannesburg: Konrad Adenauer Stiftung.

Shuma, M. (1994) 'The Case of the Matrilineal Mwera', in Tumbo-Masabo and R. Liljeström, eds, *Chelewa, Chelewa: The Dilemma of Teenage Girls*. Sweden: Nordiska Afrikainstitutet, pp. 120–32.

Simpson, A. and Heap, B. (2002) *Process Drama: A Way of Changing Attitudes.* Stockholm: Save the Children.

Sithole, J. (2002) *Afrol News,* 31 March 2002.

Sontag, S. (1988) *AIDS and Its Metaphors.* New York: Farrar, Straus & Giroux.

Spivak, G. (1988) 'Can the Subaltern Speak?', in *Marxism and the Interpretation of Culture,* ed. C. Nelson and L. Grossberg Urbana: University of Illinois Press.

Struensee, Vanessa von (2005) 'Widows, AIDS, Health, and Human Rights in Africa', see: http://www.crisisstates.com/download/forum/HIV/901widowsaids. pdf (accessed April 2007).

Swantz, M.-L. (1984) *Women in Development: A Creative Role Denied?* New York: St. Martin's Press.

Thompson, James. (2003) *Applied Theatre: Bewilderment and Beyond.* Oxford and Bern: Peter Lang.

Toolis, K. (2002 )'Killer on the Road', *The Guardian,* 3 July, see: http://www. guardian.co.uk/world/2002/jul/03/aids.kevintoolis (accessed 12 April 2010).

Turner, V. (1982) *From Ritual to Theatre: The Human Seriousness of Play.* New York: PAJ Publications.

Turner, V. (1967) *The Forest of Symbols: Aspects of Ndembu Ritual.* Ithaca, NY: Cornell University Press 1970.

Turner, Victor (1964) 'Symbols in Ndembu Ritual', in *Closed Systems and Open Minds,* ed. Max Gluckman. Edinburgh: Oliver & Boyd.

Turner, Victor ([1957] 1996) *Schism and Continuity in an African Society: A Study of Ndembu Village Life.* Oxford and Washington DC: Berg.

UNGASS *Country Progress Report: Tanzania Mainland* (2008), Dar es Salaam: Tanzania Commission for AIDS.

Van Gennep, A. (1960) *The Rites of Passage.* London: Routledge.

Vansina, J. (1985) *Oral Tradition as History.* Madison: University of Wisconsin Press.

Waal de, Alex (2006) *AIDS and Power: Why There is No Political Crisis – Yet.* London: Zed Books.

Wendo, C. (2002) 'Uganda stands firm on health spending', *The Lancet,* 360:9348 (16 December), 1847.

Wittgenstein, L. (1996) *Philosophical Investigations.* Oxford: Balckwell.

## Non-literary sources

Avert: http://www.avert.org/origin-aids-hiv.htm (accessed 15 April 2010).

*FHI/UNAIDS Best Practices in HIV/AIDS Prevention Collection* (2001), ed. Bunmi Makinwa and Mary O'Grady: http://www.fhi.org/NR/rdonlyres/e3hmq5w4o542tmtlhi66-rtwqijhfqqzgaspcwkc55f327e6dvdc5a2d5zwjdbdhhl7mgw6bprtmhip/FHIUNA IDSBestPracticesreduxenhv.pdf (accessed 9 April 2010).

National AIDS Control Programme (NACP) (2005, 2006, 2007, 2008) Surveillance Reports: http://www.nacp.go.tz/.

Ndunguru, R. (director), et.al. *Duara* (2003) film that was collectively written by students at the Fine and Performing Arts Department, University of Dar es Salaam.

Population Action International (2010) ' Fewer or More? The Real Story of Global Population': http://www.populationaction.org/Publications/Fact_Sheets/FS32/ Population_Growth.pdf (accessed 1 May 2010).

*Steps for the Future*, documentary film: http://steps.co.za/ (accessed 11 April 2010).

Tanzania AIDS Commission for AIDS (TACAIDS) (2009), Midterm Scheme (2008–12): http://www.entersoftsystems.com/tacaids/documents/NMSF%20% 202008%20-2012.pdf (accessed 25 August 2009).

UNAIDS/WHO (2004, 2005, 2006, 2007, 2008, 2009) 'Report on the global AIDS epidemic'. Geneva, see: http://www.unaids.org.

United Nations Programme on HIV/AIDS and the United Nations Development Fund for Women (UNAIDS/UNIFEM) (2010). 'Fifty-Fourth Session of the Commission on the Status of Women': http://data.unaids.org/pub/PressStat ement/2010/20100311_unaidsunifemstatementcsw54_fordistribution_rev1a_ en.pdf (accessed 1 May 2010).

UN Integrated Regional Information Networks 18 March 2002; see: http://www. aegis.com/news/irin/2002/Ir020305.html (accessed 1 May 2010).

WHO (2006) World Health Statistics 2006: (http://www.who.int/whosis/who-stat2006/en/index.html (accessed 1 May 2010).

'Widows, AIDS, Health, and Human Rights in Africa': http://www.crisisstates. com/download/forum/HIV/901widowsaids.pdf, pp. 25–6, 2005

## Interviews with individuals

Gideon Kwesigabo, Dean at Muhimbili University College of Health Sciences, Dar es Salaam, 29 May 2007.

Henry Meena, Programme Associate at UNAIDS/TACAIDS in Dar es Salaam, 21 May 2007.

Mgunga Mwa Mwenyelwa, Parapanda Lab Arts, Dar es Salaam, 7 August 2002.

Emmanuel Kazungu, Secretary General in Forum for Grassroots Organizations in Tanzania (FOGOTA), Dar es Salaam, 25 May 2007.

# Index

Abah, Oga S., 140, 143, 160n
Ahlberg, B. M., 94
AIDS
  in Africa, 1, 3, 7, 10, 16, 18, 21–2,
    26, 36, 40–1, 51–2
  in Tanzania, 3, 5, 7, 10, 16, 18,
    21–2, 26, 36, 40–1, 51–2, 72,
    81–2, 86–7, 92, 116, 124, 127,
    132, 139, 142–6
  in the world, 29–31, 33
  and health-care, 1, 24, 26, 35–9, 50,
    55, 91, 124, 136, 142, 144
  and religion, 16, 21–2, 26–8, 31, 36,
    42, 48, 51–2, 54–5, 57, 59–62, 65,
    67, 71–2, 74, 79, 86–90, 98, 109,
    118, 127, 132, 136–40
Ajzen, I., 39
anti-retroviral medicine, 3, 15, 16, 35,
    58, 68, 70, 81, 110, 132, 141
Appleton, J., 53
Arnfred, S., 31, 48
Austin, J. L., 62, 63, 64, 72, 78, 127,
    162n, 163n

Bakari, J., 160n
Banham, M., 48, 66, 156n, 168n
Barba, E., 139
Barnett, T., 35, 36, 40, 58
Barongo, G., 157n
Barthes, R., 63
Barz, G. F., 163n
Bell, C., 65
Biodun, J., 160n
Blaikie, P. M., 36
Bloch, M., 62
Boal, A., 6, 42, 45, 143, 145, 146, 148,
    156n, 161n, 162n
Boon, R., 161n
Botswana, 2, 3, 6, 36, 42, 50, 66, 67,
    70, 101
Bourgault, L., 160n, 163n
Bowling, A., 94, 104, 165n
Butler, J., 63

Byam, D. L., 44, 145, 160n, 161n
Bynum, Caroline Walker, 60

Campbell, C., 38, 40, 45, 140, 165n,
    167n
Cavell, S., 63, 162n
Clifford, J., 61, 62
Cohen-Cruz, J., 5–6, 156n
colonial issues, 6, 8, 20–1, 35, 40–1,
    46, 52, 55, 57, 65–6, 136, 139
Conner, M., 39
Coutinho, A., 167n
Crow, B., 160n

dance, 5, 11, 16–17, 25, 27, 48, 50–2,
    57, 61, 65, 70, 74, 76, 99–100,
    108, 113, 115, 119, 121, 129, 135
Dilger, H., 60–1

Easterly, W., 167n
Edmonson, L., 161n
Etherton, M., 160n
Ethiopia, 26, 71
ethnicity, 18, 20–1, 26, 35–6, 40, 54,
    60, 71, 74, 98, 134
Eyoh, Ansel, 60

Fanon, E., 146
Feldhendler, Daniel, 45
Foreman, Martin, 48
Frank, Marion, 12, 46, 68, 73, 160n,
    161n
Franko, M., 158n, 162n
Freire, P., 6, 42, 44, 45, 67, 143,
    145–46, 160n, 161n
Freudenthal, S., 39

Gausset, Q., 60
Gerholm, T., 59
gender inequality, 22, 25, 26–32, 38,
    41, 45, 53, 76, 80, 94, 100, 103–4,
    107, 112, 118, 134, 146
  and politics, 18, 42, 47, 54, 60, 118,
    120, 137–8

gender inequality – *continued*
  and prostitution, 18, 52, 83–4, 90,
    99–100, 107–18, 136
  and research, 28, 44, 88, 96, 99,
    109, 124
  and role formation, 25, 40, 48, 50,
    83, 112, 135–6
Giddens, A., 92–3
Gilbert, H., 66
Goffman, E., 64, 165n
Görgen, R., 74
Green, A. E., 64
Grimes, R. L., 61, 76
Grossberg, Lawrence, 160n
Gunderson, F., 163n

Hansson, S., 136
Harding, F., 160n
Hatar, A., 17, 42, 161n, 168n
Heap, B., 46, 140
Heggenhougen, K., 168n
Holden, S., 45
Holmdahl, B., 31
Honderich, T., 165n

Iliffe, J., 34, 35, 42, 53, 58, 60, 164n
Irobi, E., 167n

Jackson, H., 159n
Johansson, O., 162n
Jordan–Harder, B., 139, 161n

Kalipeni, E., 45
Kamlongera, C., 160n
Kasfir, N., 140
Kaunda, Kenneth, 68, 70
Kazungu, Emmanuel, 159n
Kenya, 8, 9, 53
Kerr, D., 6, 44–6, 67, 85, 139, 140,
    160n, 163n, 165n, 168n
Kidd, R., 6, 45, 140, 160n
Killewo, J., 18, 164n
Klink, M., 134, 160n
Konings, E., 31
Kwesigabo, G., 93, 134, 139, 161n,
    166n

Lange, S., 65, 74, 100, 157n, 161n
Lesotho, 42, 44, 60
Lincoln, Bruce, 60

Lugalla, J., 168n
Lutaaya, Philly, 68

Mabala, R., 74, 160n
Mandela, Nelson, 3, 68, 136, 148
Materego, G., 160n
Mazzuki, W. M. S., 127
Mbembe, A., 21
Mbizvo, Elizabeth, 144
Mda, Z., 44, 49, 160n, 161n
Mead, George H., 49
Meena, Henry, 18, 159n
Mkapa, Benjamin, 72
Mkapa, William., 36
Mlama, P., 24, 44–5, 52–5, 160n, 161n
Mlelwa, H. C., 157
music, 5, 11–12, 83
Mutembei, A. K., 35
Mwa Mwenyelwa, Mgunga, 74

Narrow, J., 94, 166n
Ndunguru, Richard, 161n
Nelson, C., 160n
*ngoma*, 5, 25, 48, 108, 119, 135
Nicholson, Helen, 125, 143
Norcross, A., 165n
Norman, P., 39
Nugent, P., 39, 58, 70, 159n
Nyanje, P., 165n
Nyoni, Frowin Paul, 45, 70, 161n

Ormrod, J. E., 39
Osofisan, Femi, 156n, 161n

Piot, Peter, 1
Plastow, J., 71, 160n, 161n
Pompêo Nogueira, M., 160n
post-colonial issues, 6, 21, 31, 40, 58,
    65–7, 119, 139–40, 146
Pritchett, James A., 162n
Putnam, Robert, 140, 167n

radio, 16, 26, 68
Rappaport, R. A., 64–5, 56, 76
Reinelt, J. G., 164n
research, 18, 20, 22–3, 28, 30, 38, 41,
    46, 57, 61
  and epidemiology, 4, 23, 27, 28, 30,
    36, 93

and fieldwork, 4, 13, 16–18, 29, 57, 61, 104
and focus group discussions, 23, 28–9, 32, 76, 79–80, 84–5, 88, 90, 92, 94–105, 108, 109, 112–13, 117–19, 125, 138, 143
and interviews, 23, 28–9, 32, 74, 90–2, 94, 104, 116–17, 125, 134, 138, 142–3
as practice-based/action research, 30–1, 48, 73, 81, 90–1, 104–5, 123–4, 126, 135–7, 140, 143
Reynolds, S., 132
Riccio, T., 161n
ritual, 5, 21, 23, 26–8, 50, 52, 55, 56–68, 74–78, 79, 82, 100, 111–12, 119, 121, 124, 147
Roach, J. R., 164n
Roth Allen, Denise, 60
Rubin, Don, 66, 71

Sabin, T. D., 159n
Salhi, Kamal, 48, 140
Schechner, Richard, 63–5, 76
Seppälä, P., 19–21, 157n
Setel, Philip W., 44, 58, 168n
Shell, R., 159n
Shuma, M., 21
Simpson, A., 46, 140
Sithole, J., 70
Sontag, Susan, 163n
South Africa, 3, 8, 36, 60, 62, 68, 96, 101

Spivak, G., 160n
Steinbock, B., 165n
Struensee, Vanessa von, 164n
Swantz, M.-L., 21, 136
Swaziland, 36, 60, 101

theatre for development (TFD), 5, 6, 12, 24–5, 41–6, 66, 119, 127, 139, 143, 146
Thompson, James, 143
Tompkins, J., 66
Toolis, K., 9, 156n
Turner, V., 25, 57, 59–61, 64–5, 67, 73, 76, 162n

Uganda, 9, 12, 18, 29, 36, 46, 51, 52, 54, 68, 70, 73, 82, 86, 93, 128

Van Gennep, A., 57, 60, 61
Vansina, J., 47

Waal, Alex de, 134
Wendo, C., 70
Whiteside, A., 35, 40, 58
Wittgenstein, L., 63

youth, 19, 21, 25–6, 47, 49–50, 54–5, 67, 71, 74–5, 81, 87–8, 97, 107, 110, 112–13, 115, 125, 141–2, 147

Zimbabwe, 36, 42, 60, 101